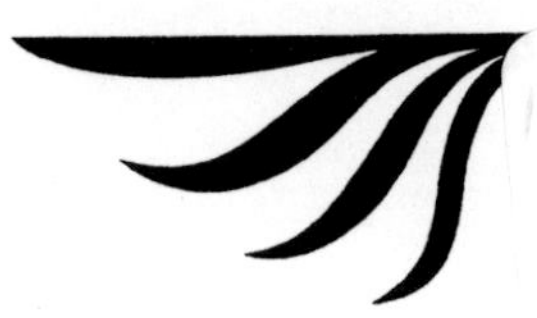

Peace Management

A clear, concise, and easy program designed to remove stress from your vocabulary

Gina Marie McKee, MSN, RN, CCRN
Associate Professor of Nursing

Jennifer Saifman, Illustrator

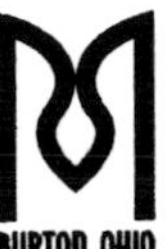

Peace management

author: Gina Marie McKee
illustrator: Jennifer Saifman

The author of this book does not dispense medical advice or prescribe the use of any technique as a form of treatment for physical or medical problems. The intent of the author is only to offer information of a general nature to help you on your quest for well-being. In the event you use any of the information in this book for yourself, which is your constitutional right, the author assumes no responsibility for your actions.

ISBN: 0-9766275-0-7

Library of Congress Control Number: 2005903253

Additional copies of this book are available at:
www.peacemanagement.info

PRINTED IN THE UNITED STATES OF AMERICA

by
Morris Publishing
3212 E. Hwy 30
Kearney, NE 68847

This book is dedicated to my son

Grant Eric Seimon

who continually challenges me to grow,
and who, because of his uncanny maturity and insights,
often ends up "raising" me.

Grant,
initially, you gave me the impetus and desire to be a successful
Peace manager.
Being a Peace manager creates
the opportunity for health and joy,
which allows me to fully experience the
blessing of watching you evolve.

With love and a deep wish for your continual Peace,
Mom

Contents

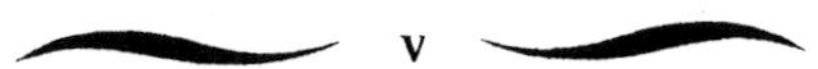

PART 3 TECHNIQUES

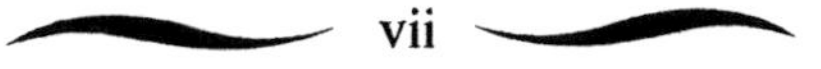

PART 4 FORMING A GROUP

PART 5 PATHOPHYSIOLOGY OF SRTRESS

PART 6 SUMMARY & FUTURE OF PEACE MANAGEMENT

Acknowledgments

With inadequately expressible gratitude to
the Universal One,
which we all are and are of

A special thank you to people who influenced me and assisted me in creating and releasing this concept and book:

My husband, Gary,
who, in addition to all his actual assistance with the book, including
countless hours of proofing and engaging
in content-driven conversations,
provides support, love, and guidance

All my nursing students,
who allowed me to experiment with them
for program development and who gave continual, valuable feedback,
and also challenged me to make abstract concepts clearer, and
clearer, and clearer

All my patients (and patients in general),
who inspired the creation of the book

All the people whom I initially viewed as difficult,
but who actually ended up being my best teachers in my progress
toward becoming a Peace manager

My revered teachers,
including Jerry Leitz, Karl, and Michael

Meryl F. Soto-Schwartz, Ph.D.
whose insights and assistance went far beyond her role as the
copy editor

Jennifer Saifman
illustrator extraordinaire
and for assuming the role of artistic designer for this project

James Landis, M.D., Ph.D., CSCS,
who initially reviewed the chapter on the
"Pathophysiology of Stress," but due to his passion for teaching and
health was asked to co-author this section

Philip Roskos,
Professor of Chemistry, Lakeland Community College,
for all your insight as a scientist who has a love of
philosophy and people

content reviewers:

Marc Finney
Mike Krupa
Pat Cyrgalis
Lori Aerietta
"Auntie LoLo"
Joe Mondello
all of my students

final draft review:
Kathleen L. Kuhar, RN
Gary L. McKee

everyone at Morris Publishing,
with special gratitude for
the talented individuals in the art department and Bob Wallace

Marci Bulman,
of Marci's Hair on the Square,
for providing professional services in a professional manner

Michael Corbley,
of Michael Corbley Photography, for his artistic creation
through photography

Kim, Jackie, and Kyle Schroeder,
for constant inspiration and support

everyone who provided peripheral support, including
Brian and Hany at Fullcircle Promotions, Inc.
Don and Suzette Miller, Jeff Brunty, Jessica Novak
Madeline S. Sharp (Aunt Maddy)

Peace Management: Concept Not Completed

Preface

April 9, 1999

I sit here at my computer, pulling my thoughts together, at the end of my shift at the hospital. Something very significant happened tonight. Tonight was the first night I realized that the techniques I had been using to maintain Peace could be transformed into a program that others could integrate into their lives as well.

From March 1997 until December 1998, I struggled through a very emotional and stressful divorce. I am sure there are many people who can relate to the chaos that is created by a divorce. As the divorce progressed, I witnessed the toll the stress was taking on not only me, but my family as well. It became clear that the stress did not improve the situation or circumstances. In fact, the only consequence of stress was a negative impact on those involved. I realized we needed something very different. I devoted a great deal of time and attention to figuring out how to help myself and my family. Soon after, I began sharing these ideas with friends and co-workers. We all began shifting the way we experienced things. This approach to well-being is what soon came to be known as "Peace management."

During my shift at work tonight, I witnessed a patient and her husband react enthusiastically to my ideas. I now realize that I need to expand and refine these techniques and develop them into a program that could be used by the vast majority of people.

Peace management goes far beyond the 80's buzzword, stress management and the 90's notion of anger management. Peace management is a whole way of being, of existing. *It truly is life altering.*

Tonight, as I was standing at the bedside of my patient, Shelly, while her doctor, a neurologist, was sharing the results of her tests, the light went on for me. This patient needed to internalize a very potent plan, and I might have the answer for her. She was a 39 year old female of Spanish descent. She had a clipping of an aneurysm in her brain ten years ago. Several years following the procedure, she developed seizure activity. She became very fearful about the seizures. At that time, she found they seemed to be caused by stressful events. Following that initial period, her seizures became very well controlled by her medication; she went several years without a seizure. Then a couple of months ago, she had some life changing events that caused her a great deal of stress. She became fearful that her seizures would return. Following the resurfacing of this fear, she began having episodes of passing out at work, at home, in stores, wherever she was experiencing stress peaks.

Because of Shelly's history with seizures, everyone assumed that the episodes were seizures. Her neurologist, who had strong intuitive feelings that these episodes were her reaction to stress, began a comprehensive battery of tests in an effort to rule out any real pathological cause. Not surprisingly, everything came back "normal." This is where I came into the picture. I entered the room with the doctor, which is normal practice when informative interactions are expected to ensue. What most would perceive as good news, (normal results) was actually devastating to the patient and her husband. They both obviously hoped for good news, but if there was something that was wrong that could be fixed by "the right combination of medications" Shelly could be back on her way to

* *names and identifying details have been altered throughout this book to protect the privacy of my patients, students, friends, and relatives.*

health. Now, both Shelly and her husband feared there was no "quick fix." They both felt she could not possibly control the stress that precipitated the episodes of passing out. Therefore, they concluded, when the stress appeared, Shelly would pass out.

Shelly's husband said that he has done everything he could think of to relieve her stress, from doing the household bill-paying and disciplining their daughters, to helping her plan ways to reduce stress at work. None of these had really helped, and the couple didn't want to consider anti-anxiety medications. I could feel their helplessness and their deflated hope. The doctor, in an attempt to remedy this, said "there are good ways to manage stress." I saw their spirits sink even further. I was already involved in the conversation, because we were talking about discharge planning, so I said "as part of our discharge planning, I am going to work with you on 'Peace management'."

It is a philosophy I have only recently solidified, but it fit in so appropriately with this patient that I had to share it with her, ready or not. It was the actual birth and delivery of this new term. I saw a resuscitation of Shelly and her husband's spirits. I knew I was on to something. I realized that the concept that has become the way I live and that my friends and family are trying to incorporate might become the most valuable tool of my career.

Following my statement that I would work on "Peace management" with Shelly, I sensed a relief in the physician, who also witnessed the new spark and sense of hope in his patient. At this time though, I would like to provide you with a sense of what was going on in my mind as I left the room.

> I essentially said, "Oh sh _ _, that family is depending on me and I don't know exactly what it is that I am going to say. I have ideas swirling around in my mind, but I have never presented this in a formal way before. And it certainly never had a name."

Well, my shift was very busy and I was not able to get back into the patient's room during my shift. (Luckily this bought me some time.) However, I told them I would be back later. After my shift was over, I entered Shelly's room, gave Shelly and her husband my undivided attention, and began discussing the concept with them. The words flowed out as if someone else, who knew what she was talking about, was speaking. I had to stop every few minutes and just allow myself to take it all in. I must say the level of development of the ideas and the amount of information I presented even overwhelmed me at times. The patient's husband lit up. He said, "this is exactly what we need. This is what I have been trying to communicate to her but didn't have a framework for explaining it." He told me he was an engineer and "thinks in a certain way." He had "needed a framework to try and tie it all together. This is exactly what I have been searching for." After Shelly and her husband said all the cliché niceties like "you are an angel sent by God" and "there was a reason you were sent to care for my wife tonight," we got down to the real work. That is when we got into the specific concepts that are the content of this book.

I have been a practicing nurse in intensive care settings for over 20 years. I also teach nursing. I have taught at a very prestigious university and at a very spiritually oriented Catholic college. I currently teach nursing at a well respected, local community college. In this program, I am currently working with several women and men who are creating their careers, within what many of us would label as stressful life circumstances. Some of my students are single mothers, many with two or more children, working to pay bills and provide health insurance while struggling through the demands of a very tough and rigorous curriculum. I have some students from other countries who have had to temporarily leave their families to acquire an education that will allow them to provide for their families in the long term. I have some students who were drawn to nursing because they have a child with chronic illness. I have people going through divorces that are turning to a career that will give their lives a sense of purpose. And that is just the beginning of the list of issues that many of my students face as they live their lives and keep their heads above water. My students and my role as an instructor provide the perfect metaphorical "classroom" for me to assist people with incorporating Peace management into their lives.

Throughout my career as a nurse, I have always worked to become a very skilled clinician, but I have frequently become frustrated by my limitations. Technology can only do so much. I had always hoped and prayed that I could actually be a part of my patients' healing. Although I prayed for that gift, I wasn't sure if it could ever be realized or how it could happen. I have heard time and time again that one's prayers are always answered, to meet one's deepest, heart-felt desire. The actual result may not look as we had it pictured, but the prayer will be answered. It is now very clear to me that there is a great need for mental and emotional healing that will lead to physical healing. I may not heal in the traditional sense of the word, but I feel that Peace management could be the tool that leads to healing for many people in need.

November 2003

Okay, enough is enough! It is time to sit down and get my ideas on paper. I have been living with them for 7 years now - watching them, practicing them, teaching them, evaluating them - knowing the message had to get out, but allowing fear and doubt to block this work. As you can see from the previous date, Peace management even had a name back in 1999. This information needs to be presented. It is a concept that has proven to have immense value.

The biggest block to work on this book was my own self analysis of my exponential growth as I practice Peace management in my own life. I say to myself, "I am growing so fast; how can I sit down mid-growth and write about it. I need to 'get there' and then look back and present it." How silly, because in my heart I know there is no real end or "getting there." It really is an on-going evolution. So my plan, at this point, is to share what I know at present and just resign myself to there being a sequel (or 2 or 3). Okay, time to move on!

What is Peace management? It is a way to live life from a place of Peace amidst a set of circumstances that present chaos, stress, confusion, fear, and isolation. I am not alone. And neither are you. We have good company. I know it from the hundreds to thousands of dialogues I have engaged in since the concept of Peace management came into my life.

I would like to comment on two other areas that affect the style of this book. The first is that I am not a psychologist, a sociologist, or a theologian. Therefore, I offer no expertise in these areas, even though some areas may feel incomplete due to the lack of inclusion of these perspectives. My expertise is in nursing (which has provided an understanding of people and their situations), education, and Peace management. Therefore, these are the only areas I can speak on from authority, expertise, and experience. I must also note, there is no scientific research supporting the positive effects of Peace management on health at this point, since it is a relatively new concept. However, there is a multitude of anecdotal stories to support the benefits.

The second comment relates to the framework for this book. I am very comfortable with my spirituality, but I did not want this to be a spiritually based book, for fear of alienating a large segment of population. It would be a disservice to this topic and the people I am trying to reach if I let my personal beliefs interfere with someone accessing Peace management. This was a tough one for me. I didn't want to turn off individuals who are coming from a secular orientation, and I did not want people of a spiritual orientation to feel something important was missing. You will probably identify both flavors throughout this book. I apologize if it interferes with the flow and meaning. I simply ask you to take the specific information and place it into a framework that works for you. We're in this together. This allows for creativity on both our parts.

I choose not to use the abbreviation PM at this point. This idea is too new. I feel people need to hear the term "Peace management" over and over as a concept, until our society really begins to internalize it, until it becomes the way we automatically act.

My hope is that the contents of this book create a shift in the way you experience life. My hope is that it is a full life, filled with various experiences, but that it is experienced from a point and perspective of Peace. I live Peace and witness the shift in the people whom I directly counsel in this area. Best wishes on your journey of experiencing Peace.

Part 1:

Raising Consciousness

1 THE NEED FOR PEACE MANAGEMENT

Very early in my nursing career, I became aware of something that had altered the way I view illness and disease. In both of my roles, as a clinician (a nurse at the bedside) in Intensive Care Units and Emergency Departments, and as an educator, working with patients with diabetes and heart disease, something became crystal clear to me. It caused me to watch this phenomenon closely throughout my career, in every encounter I had with a patient.

I was only 22 years old when I became a registered nurse, as green as they come with very minimal life experience, having lived a very sheltered childhood. However, looking back, this is what allowed me to have a clean slate as I entered my career. I did not come to nursing and patients with any preconceived ideas or judgment. I took what patients told me at face value and was able to clearly recognize and identify patterns.

My patients must sense this lack of judgment and my genuine interest in their health and healing. They trust me. Therefore, they are very willing to open up and share their deepest, darkest, and scariest stories with me. Over time, I came to realize that most of the people suffering from a serious disease or illness shared something in common. That "thing" was stress. Either they lived a life full of several stressors (a very "charged" way of living) or had experienced one major event that created their intense stress.

Unfortunately, patients would develop a disease, experience physical pain, or have a "flare-up" of a pre-existing chronic illness. Almost without fail! And believe me, since Peace management has become my baby and my path, I have been delving deeply into my patients' history.

Before the advent of insurance companies creating limits on hospital admissions, diabetic patients could be admitted with a diagnosis of "uncontrolled blood sugar." During the portion of my career when I was a Diabetic Educator, I came to know my patients very well. I would work with them on an out-patient basis, and I would also be involved with their care while they were hospitalized. As part of my assessment, I would ask them about events that precipitated their admission. Almost 100% had experienced a major life stressor (the only exception being the flu or infection). As you will see later, an elevation of blood sugar (and this is the problem for diabetics) is one of the ways the body responds to stress. And believe it or not, this is actually one of the *least* harmful responses the body has to stress.

I carried my inquiry from working with patients with diabetes to groups of patients with various other medical diagnoses. I found a strong correlation between stress and various other chronic illnesses, especially diseases that are categorized as autoimmune (the body attacking itself) in nature or that have an autoimmune component. This coincides with current research findings. I believe that in the future, research will actually prove a much stronger link between stress and autoimmune disease. This will demonstrate that stress is a more frequent etiology (cause) of some of the disease processes we now have. A current study that is trying to demonstrate a link between autoimmune factors and disease has captured my attention because it relates to my specialty in nursing. Researchers are now trying to identify a link between autoimmunity and congestive heart failure.

What most of you also realize is that stress does not just correlate with chronic illness (an illness that has a long duration and progresses slowly), but acute illness (an illness that has a rapid onset and a brief course) as well. Many people get the cold, flu, or other infections during periods of stress. Stress and negative emotions affect the immune system (the disease fighting or resisting system). Part 5 of the book provides a more in depth discussion on the pathophysiologic effects of stress, or the role it plays in the body. It is at the end of the book because it is really optional reading for those seeking to master Peace management. We do not need to understand the cell level effects of stress to know it is harmful. However, there will be some readers who need extra convincing that stress really is detrimental to their health and well being before they will be willing to make any life changes. I have included Part 5 in this book for them or anyone else who simply is curios.

I envision a world where everyone lives life from a place of Peace. I realize this book will be read by people with various interest levels, education levels, and resistance/acceptance levels. My deep desire is that this Peace management reaches and affects everyone. I know some of you need to approach things from a total, deep understanding. If you fall into this category, you may want to jump to Part 5 first. Grab yourself a cup of tea and a quiet corner. You will be in for some heavy-duty material.

I became very saddened as I did my literature search for Part 5 of the book. There were thousands of articles about the ill effects of stress and its link to disease. There were only a few articles on peace and a few more research articles looking at the effects of stress management programs on disease reduction. This link between stress and illness has been known for quite a while. We are missing the boat! It is time to take our awareness to the next step and *prevent* disease and illness by addressing its root causes: stress, anger, and other negative emotions.

If you look around you, you will find frequent references to the fact that stress adversely affects health and well-being. You will see testimony to this connection frequently. Professionals from various backgrounds attest to it. I was made aware of the popular discourse on this subject during one day when I felt I was bombarded from various areas. Three examples from that day follow:

- I called in to the Cleveland Clinic (a world renowned hospital where celebrities and dignitaries often choose to be treated) to talk to someone in the research department. I was placed on what they call a meet-me line. The Clinic's phone system plays various advertising and education pieces while callers wait. The first one I heard talked about the "harmful effects of stress on the body," then proceeded to give tips on stress management techniques.

- The second example occurred during a nursing faculty meeting at the college. We were discussing the initiation of various entrance exams. A faculty member noted that most companies who make these tests are now including a stress level profile. They have found that students who "handle stress better" are more successful in nursing school.

- The third stress-related discussion I heard during that same day was in an unusual place for me. I do not watch TV with any regularity. In fact, we lost our TV after a lightening strike and did not purchase a new one for six months. The only channel I watch is the Travel Channel (nothing stressful there!). I turned on the TV to that channel and they had on one of those infomercials. I was ready to turn off the TV when I heard the word "stress". The infomercial was promoting a product that reduces cortisol levels. The physician on TV was talking about the release of cortisol during stress. He described the linkage between cortisol and certain types of weight gain. He said his product not only relieves stress but also reduces weight. I can not verify this, but I did find it very interesting.

I will frequently use the word stress as the opposite of Peace in this book. I use the word "stress" as a catch-all word, but I want you to know that any negative emotion can have the same detrimental effect on the body. During a CPR class, my instructor drove home another very important point. She was discussing the risk factors for heart disease. Most people are accustomed to hearing about the danger triad: smoking, high blood pressure, and high cholesterol. However, she drew our attention to a topic receiving more interest and attention. She said that researchers and cardiologists are identifying the strong link that exists between heart disease and a specific personality trait (and it is not the previously touted Type A personality). It is the *person who is filled with anger and hostility*. Many participants in the class seemed surprised. Not me! I can verify it in my own cardiac nursing practice.

The word "disease" can be broken down into "dis - ease", or without ease. Florence Scovel Shinn, the grandmother of metaphysics, in 1925, in *The Game of Life and How to Play It* (p. 27) states "every disease is caused by a mind not at ease."

One of the major dangers of stress is the downward spiral:

stress → disease → stress about the disease → worsening of disease

In other words, stress leads to disease or illness. This creates additional stress for the person, which then leads to worsening of the disease, and so on, and so on, and so on. People can actually have a total preoccupation with their disease, which places them in almost constant stress. This is a gradual downward spiral. Peace management can break this spiraling effect. If the spiral is not broken, premature death is a common result. It is never too late to learn Peace management.

Why Peace management? What I have come to see is that the 80's fashion of teaching "stress management" (and I was a part of that, teaching it to new employees at a community hospital) and the 90's focus on "anger management", in terms of being beneficial to your health, is actually **TOO LATE**!!! These techniques, in a sense, allow people to experience the stress or anger and then implement techniques of management, to come back to their baseline. Credit must be given to the originators of stress and anger management. It was a start, but these two approaches have two shortcomings.

The first problem is that if you allow yourself to experience stress or anger, even for a brief time, it triggers the stress response in the body. This means that the harmful chemicals have already been released in your body to do the damage. The second problem is that it only works to get you back to your baseline. Your "baseline" is your usual state of being, in day-to-day life. And for many of us, that baseline is not desirable. I can attest to that in my own life. My current baseline, because of Peace management is much calmer, more peaceful, and more joyful. Peace is not simply the absence of fear, worry, anger, or stress. It is a whole way of being.

Stress management and anger management techniques are **TOO LATE**!!!!! Peace management builds on the insights of those who pioneered stress management and anger management, but it is proactive rather than reactive. Because it prevents rather than merely responds to stress, it more effectively enables people to achieve health and joy.

THE PROCESS

2

If you have read this far, you have already entered the first phase of the process—*Raising Consciousness.* This simply means that the need for Peace management has come to the forefront of your mind. It *is* an issue, and one worth your attention. It is time to look at Peace management in more depth, and to identify the role and significance that stress and anger play in your life.

This program is called Peace management because the goal is for you to eventually maintain your Peace in all of life's circumstances, with room for occasional slip-ups. The Peace needs to be valued, protected, and maintained throughout your daily living. This takes management skills. Some of the phrases used to define management are:

to have charge of
to do what one wishes, especially by skill
to conduct or direct affairs
to succeed in handling matters

The word "management" is used frequently (stress management, anger management, business management, nursing management, etc.) because it connotes directing the way the outcome is achieved, that things do not happen in a haphazard way. That is exactly what I am suggesting should happen with your Peace. Your goal is to maintain your natural state of Peace. There are outside circumstances that will try to rob it, yet you will remain in the driver's seat and manage and maintain your Peace. It will take awareness, skill, and various strategies to learn how to regularly integrate Peace into your new way of life. Once you experience Peace, you will want to protect it. You are the gatekeeper of your Peace.

While reading this book, you may sense repetition and redundancy. It is actually an intended strategy. This book incorporates a form of mind-training. Not an easy feat. Therefore it will require that you become inundated with a type of information and that I repeatedly present it with slight twists. Different things click for different people. Something presented one way to an individual will lack meaning, but in another context can be a life altering idea.

I have found that for some individuals, the idea of Peace management can bring about change in an epiphany-like fashion. They hear the concept and realize that this is the framework that answers their frustrations. They hear it, take off, and do their own work. The next time I see them, they tell me that "from the last time I saw you, I totally turned around my life. I made a choice in that moment for Peace and never turned back."

Some of you will need to try on various strategies until one clicks for you. And like the first group, once you genuinely experience Peace as a way of life, there will be no turning back—you will never choose stress or anger again. Primitive responses may kick in and give you a "charge" occasionally, but even then, you learn to recognize what is happening and you will be able to bring yourself back to baseline quickly. For me, at this point, when I do experience those rare moments of stress, I need about three deep breaths. It's as if the stress never pulsed through my system. My goal is to eventually accomplish this with one deep breath!

I will warn you that as you read the first two sections of this book, you may experience a bit of frustration (and you can believe it is not my intention to create a stressful situation). Many who have read this material say they wanted to "get right to the work of being a Peace manager." Trust me on this one: going right to the techniques would not serve you well. The process of becoming a Peace manager is *your* process. You will find that as you read this book and have a heightened consciousness about Peace, stress, and anger you will begin the process of self exploration. This is vital to the process.

If you start right in on techniques and strategies, it will become a mechanical process, not one that originates from the depth of your being. Believe me, if you are reading the book, you have started the process; *you don't need to know "how to do it" to begin.* Please see that immersing yourself in the concept is the way to begin.

When I start my nursing students in this program, I purposefully give them only the first few sections of the book. Yes, I do hear their frustrations of "wanting more NOW." However, what actually happens is much more valuable. They cannot keep reading, therefore they begin many discussions with their peers in school. They tell me they have called their best friend or sister-in-law to discuss the ideas and they photocopy chapters for their mother or neighbor. They begin using the vocabulary in this book. I revel in hearing this! They are on their way. They are making Peace management part of their consciousness and their essence.

We are accustomed to instant gratification. We get a hamburger at a fast food restaurant in 45 seconds, we have instant access to information via the Internet, we get macaroni and cheese in the microwave in seconds. That may be what causes the frustration with wanting Peace NOW. I am sorry, but it doesn't come in a bottle. You have to create it. Think of it as a masterpiece in process. It will be well worth the wait and the work involved.

You will soon realize that this process is simple but not easy. It is hard to change old habits and patterns, but once you experience it, you value it. Once you value it, you protect it. Once you protect it, it becomes your way of existence.

<u>The actual process of utilizing Peace management is:</u>

- raising consciousness
- examining yourself—understanding when you are stressed or angry and the specific effects on your body
- valuing and protecting Peace
- employing a strategy
- evaluating its effectiveness
- trying a new strategy
- evaluating its effectiveness, and so on
- enjoying Peace

An important concept and phrase I would like to introduce is the "*charge*." It will be used throughout the book, because it is the way you will monitor yourself and your progress when implementing Peace management. The "charge" is the effect or feeling in your body, in response to the negative emotion. Each person must identify how the stressor effects them in the short term. Some possibilities to look for as you try to analyze your own response are:

◊ tightening of any muscles
◊ a "knot" or "butterflies" in the stomach
◊ heart pounding
◊ different breathing patterns (holding breath for short periods of time)
◊ erratic movements of arms
◊ a lump in the throat
◊ hives
◊ a lack of mental clarity
◊ tightening around the mouth
◊ flaring of the neck muscles
◊ flaring of the nostrils
◊ repetitive movements (finger tapping, leg shaking, etc.)
◊ nervous tics
◊ clouded thinking
◊ perspiration
◊ burning from acid reflux

The word "charge" will become a regular part of your vocabulary; you will find yourself uttering it frequently as you move toward becoming an effective Peace manager. I frequently do a "charge-check" with myself, family, friends, and students.

Why do you experience a charge? You are experiencing an emotion. Let's back up one step further. What is an emotion? Let's back it another step, then move through the process.

Stress reactions start with a "negative" thought. A thought is your idea, judgment, or interpretation of a situation; something that happens in your mind. As you will see later, this is actually in your control, and will be the heart of Peace management. The next part is out of your control (and this is why control of the thought will take on such significance). What happens next is the response of the Autonomic Nervous System and Neuroendocrine System and the resulting feeling of doom, anger, or stress that it causes. This is what we call an emotion. So in a nut shell, an *emotion* is a thought coupled with the physical feeling you have from your Autonomic Nervous System's response to the thought.

Your Autonomic Nervous System is also called the *involuntary* nervous system. You do have a *voluntary* nervous system. This is the part of your nervous system that responds voluntarily to your direction. If I want to reach for a cup, my nervous system tells my muscles to move, whereas the involuntary system is just that—involuntary. It puts together the messages and response at a very subtle level. You don't tell your heart rate to get faster, or your body to release chemicals. All this happens without your conscious direction. But this is the part of the nervous system that creates the feeling of the emotion. This is what we will call the "charge."

The training that will be presented in this book will focus on *maintaining Peace as a way of eliminating the charge in the body* or eliminating the negative emotion and its effect on the body through control of the mind.

When you first begin labeling your negative emotions, you will probably categorize them in a few broad categories, namely stress, anger, and fear. You will next begin to refine your definitions and terminology and more accurately identify the subtle emotional differences. This next level might include such terms as

- resentment
- guilt
- doubt
- helpless
- hopeless
- frustration
- anxiety
- regret
- sadness
- insecurity
- vulnerability
- overwhelmed
- jealousy
- fear

Some say that there are only two real emotions: love and fear. For the sake of Peace management, it doesn't matter what you label the negative emotion, as long as you can identify it as a negative emotion and identify the "charge." We will go through the process of accurately labeling emotions, because labeling assists you with getting in touch with the vague state you may feel as stress.

I want to be very clear early on: Peace management is not about denying your feelings. That would be repression. This is not healthy and will not lead to Peace. Neither is Peace management about being the strong, silent type (if you are aware of negative emotions and hiding them from others). Hiding emotions is not emotionally healthy either. People who do so are not at Peace. This is about something very different. It is finding your Peace and then managing it. This book explains how to do just that.

Okay, here comes the teacher in me. The next section is your first homework assignment. I joke about its name, but homework is the only way to really begin integrating the information, not simply learning *about* it. Peace management can stay an academic concept for you or you can chose to make it a way of life. To change habits or behaviors they must be worked on, tried on for size, and lived. You can choose to follow the exercise to the letter or you can just do it as a mental exercise, taking yourself through the paces without putting pen to paper. In these exercises, when I am working with students, I actually call what many would refer to as an "activity" a "catalyst". This is because the exercises are intended to bring about a change. Well, go ahead and get started. Don't worry, I won't be grading you, spelling doesn't count, and there is no due date.

Exercise (A):

Raising Consciousness

Goals for this section:

- Raise your awareness of the stress, anger, and other negative emotions currently in your life
- Raise awareness that Peace is an alternate choice to stress or anger
- Identify the negative effects that stress creates in the body
- Identify these negative effects as a "charge" in the body

Activity A:

Observe yourself throughout the day. Identify the feelings you call stress and anger.

List the effects on your body as you are experiencing these feelings. Pay special attention to your breath, the tension of your muscles, and the feeling in your stomach area.

Effects in body during stress:	Effects in body during anger:
•	•
•	•
•	•
•	•

List the other negative emotions you experience:

1. ______________________ 5. ______________________

2. ______________________ 6. ______________________

3. ______________________ 7. ______________________

4. ______________________ 8. ______________________

Activity B:

Identify the relationship between stress/anger and your health. Begin to observe others and notice the relationship in them.

- In the past, stress has caused the following health problems for me:

- I have noticed that when I am stressed:

- Friends and family members that have less than optimal health (rather sickly) experience these forms of stress in their lives:

- Friends and family members that have a high level of well being and health experience these forms of stress in their lives:

The conclusions I draw are:

Part 2:

Valuing & Protecting Peace

3

I AM THE GATEKEEPER OF MY PEACE

A mental picture of a gatekeeper helps you remember that you are the person who has the control of your Peace. A gatekeeper is a person who controls passage through the gate. This metaphor encourages you to realize that Peace is something you value and that you will protect. Being a gatekeeper means protecting your Peace and not allowing anyone or anything to rob you of that Peace.

The second step in Peace management is *valuing* Peace. Closely connected to the concept of valuing is *protecting.* You can identify what people value by the fervor with which they protect it. You can always tell the people who value their cars when you are in a parking lot of a mall or the grocery store. They park in the last row or last spot, or take up two spots so that no one can park next to them and accidentally damage their car.

Believe it or not, this is exactly what I am talking about. You must first value Peace before it becomes something that you will protect with every fiber in your body.

Okay, how does this happen? Well, the only way is to have first hand experience at maintaining your Peace during a situation that would normally cause stress, anger, or any other negative emotion. If you can't experience Peace on your own, you cannot authentically support it. This is the second part of the Peace management process. Once you experience it you will value it. This will then make you willing to practice it and work on it. It will become "the way you are." It will become the style of your existence, your essence. You will have an opportunity to *value* Peace in the exercise following this chapter

Initially, the exercise is actually like a game. It allows you to experiment with a playful attitude. During this exercise, you will not feel like you are risking anything, including the loss of old patterns, even if the old patterns were counter-productive or downright harmful. We have a vested interest in developing patterns and following these patterns. Patterns allow us a certain level of comfort. In this exercise, you are simply trying Peace management on for size. See if it fits!

One aspect of valuing Peace involves feeling the immediate benefits of Peace management. The flip side of valuing Peace relates to the awareness of the toxicity that takes place in the absence of Peace. Without yet calling it "toxic" in the first exercise, you began this awareness when you identified the negative effects of stress and anger. I believe that by labeling these effects with the harsh word "toxic" you will more easily engage in the practice of valuing and protecting Peace.

Using the "Gatekeeper" philosophy is one of the easiest ways to help you maintain and protect your Peace. It is something I still use, almost in a joking manner, now that it really is so integrated into my being. My friends are also at the point that they joke with me. One friend in particular, who also happens to be a co-worker, will whisper in my ear at the beginning of what is anticipated to be a stressful meeting or interaction, "I am the Gatekeeper of my Peace." We chuckle and actually take a deep breath together. It is an easy mantra to remind yourself to stay in a place of Peace.

Exercise (B):

Valuing Peace / Gatekeeper

Goals for this section:

- Experience the benefits of acting from a place of Peace
- Identify the toxicity that arises when Peace is not present in your interactions
- Observe the toxicity that is occurring during your "quiet times" when those quiet times are not experienced as Peace
- Recognize the value of Peace
- Make a commitment to yourself that you will protect your Peace
- View yourself as the Gatekeeper of your Peace

Activity A:

Write down one situation which either

- occurs on a regular basis that causes you stress or anger (example: your spouse's attitude or actions when he/she comes home from work)
- or a stressful situation that only happens occasionally but that you know will be coming up in the near future (examples: a visit from someone, confronting a boss).

Briefly, describe this situation:

What do you usually feel during these interactions? (What is the "charge" or the effect in your body?)

Now, take a moment to make a conscious choice that you are not going to allow stress, anger, or any other negative emotion to enter the picture.

In your handwriting, write out the situation in which you will practice valuing Peace:

my example:

The next time I talk to the secretary in my doctor's office, I choose to come from a place of Peace.

your example:

The next time I ______________________________________

____________________________________, I choose to come from

a place of Peace.

Now devise your plan to make this happen. Here are some suggestions:

- view the situation as a play and yourself as an actress/actor
- view the other person from a point of pure compassion
- simply see it as an experiment

example:

I might choose to come from a place of compassion and tell myself that the secretary might not get the support she needs to do her job well

or

I might choose to pretend to be an actor who has the job of talking calmly to a hostile, overworked secretary. I do not need her assistance. I am simply the actor who has the role of talking to her. There is no emotional attachment to the situation.

It doesn't matter what approach you take at this point, you just need to take a situation that normally causes you stress or anger and do it *one time* from a place of Peace.

Now, take a moment to visualize and "play out" in your mind experiencing this situation while coming from a place of Peace.

Now, do it!
Be sure not to act phony.
Be genuine in this attempt, knowing it is the healthy way to do things.

Once you have had a chance to try out your experiment, write down your reaction when you came from a place of Peace:

- how did you feel?

- how did the other person/people respond?

- what was not there? (The charge)

Summarize how this exercise went for you:

Do you see the value of Peace?

Activity B:

Turn off the car radio this week, while you are driving, during periods when no one else is in the car, or set aside some other time that you are alone.

While you are in these quiet times, notice what occupies your thoughts. Periodically catch yourself in thought. Identify and analyze your thoughts. Are any of your thoughts creating any negative emotion during this quiet time?

Some of my negative thoughts are:

My emotions during these thoughts are:

Can you identify the above emotions as the source of your "charge"?

Be true to yourself – do you want Peace?

Are you willing to protect it?

Are you willing to give away the power to someone or something else and allow them to rob your Peace?

A TWO-TIERED CHOICE

4

Whenever you interact with others, or simply live life, there are choices on how to proceed and what to do. In relation to implementing Peace management, it is part of a two-tiered choice. The *first tier* relates to the "how." It is the decision to come from a place of Peace or to come from a place that lacks Peace. Therefore, before you choose what you will do, you must choose how you will do it. You choose to maintain your Peace through the rest of the process. It is a choice!

The *second tier* relates to the "what." It is what you will think, say, or do. It is independent of the first tier. It involves the specific *thoughts* you will have, the *words* you will choose to use, or the *actions* you will take. And there is a choice here, too. You are not a mindless robot who is set on "automatic" and programmed to think, speak, and act in a certain way.

Living in this world, your life is almost a constant stream of thinking, speaking, or doing. Your goal will be to gradually have longer periods of time where your mind experiences stillness, but currently, this constant stream of thoughts, words, and actions is a fact of your existence. Therefore, the concept of the two-tiered choice becomes magnified.

I must thank one of my nursing students, Laura, who helped me refine the way I present this concept. When I first began teaching Peace management, I did not call it a two-tiered choice, yet I would present Peace as a consciousness choice you must first make, before anything else.

In one of my group sessions, I gave the participants an exercise to promote the second step of the Peace management program: "Valuing Peace." I had them report back to me on their observations and experiences. Laura stated she liked the idea, but had a difficult time. The situation she chose to practice "Valuing Peace" centered around bedtime preparation of her children. She said, "I just can't turn off the caring or 'being the mom,' making sure they are all in bed on time to get enough rest on a school night."

Wow, that was an educational 2 x 4 across my forehead! I didn't realize that something that I take for granted was not clear to people just learning to practice Peace management. I somehow did not communicate that the choice had two tiers. Something that I had said led her to believe that to have Peace, you must not take a stand in a situation; you must take an inactive role. That is very far from the truth.

Now I make sure the concept of a two tiered choice is very clear and a well-developed concept in a Peace manager's mind. I would not want anyone to avoid practicing Peace management out of a concern that they must remain inactive. Peace management does not intend to encourage complacency or apathy. I now say, "I am far from what you would call a zombie, or one who just goes through life simply going through the motions." I have always described myself as someone who approaches life with gusto and cherishes all the experiences (yes, the lessons too) that life has to offer me. I attempt to live life to its fullest and experience the richness of every moment. I live life fully, while being a very successful Peace manager.

Peace management is the first part of a two tiered process.

This book assists you with learning about and embracing the first tier, which then sets the stage for implementing the second tier.

Let me illustrate how Laura applied this concept. Let's take the "bedtime for kids" example that Laura chose. Laura's experience was that this was normally a very stressful time of the day for her. I am not sure what occurred exactly, but I can guess that there might have been some yelling, some tears, repeating herself seventeen times before the children began the bedtime ritual. Once she decided to use this situation to try Peace, she had *two* choices to make.

The first choice (the "how"): will I be a mom who is coming from a place of Peace tonight or will stress/anger be my mode of operation?

The second choice (the "what"): is what will I do? These are called the "action choices." This choice is not specifically guided by the Peace management techniques but examples will be provided to illustrate the second tier.

In the first tier, *Laura chose to come from a place of Peace*. We discussed four possibilities that she could employ in the second tier (the action choice). The four options we chose were:

1. Say the same words and do the same things she does every night.
2. Have the children become a part of the decision making about bedtime.
3. Entice them to go to bed without a struggle.
4. Praise them for other things they did right that night and tell them that she hopes things will go as smoothly at bedtime tonight (to plant the seed).

I offered suggestions for the action choice, but it is of no concern in the Peace management process. Any one of these choices on how to handle the situation can be done from a place of Peace or from one of stress and anger. I cannot really offer expert advice on the action choice. I am not a child psychologist, I am just an experienced mom who drew on my own successes and failures to come up with some basic examples for action choices. The second tier of the choice is something Laura will have to develop on her own, obtain from a professional in the area, or another experienced mom.

As far as Peace management is concerned, ***choosing Peace is the most important part of the equation***, not the action itself. Laura can still look like a mom, sound like a mom, and act like a mom. There need not be any difference on the outside. The change occurs on the inside: there is an absence of "charge" and a feeling of Peace.

You will clearly see how this plays out when you apply this two-tiered concept to your own life situations. Let's take a few more examples to assist in applying this concept:

Dilemma	**First Tier: "how"**	**Second Tier: "what"**
My adult child asked if he could move back home after his divorce.	I can chose to come from a place of Peace or to come from a lack of Peace during the decision making process.	I can let him move back in. or I can tell him that he can not move back in.
My spouse does not spend much time with the family.	I can chose to come from a place of Peace or come from a lack of Peace when I think about this situation.	I can think about approaching him about this. or I can think about ignoring it. or I can think about having the kids directly ask him for time they would like to spend with him, and I can do the same. or countless other options.

Dilemma	First Tier: "how"	Second Tier: "what"
I purchased an appliance that doesn't work as promised.	I can chose to come from a place of Peace or come from a lack of Peace during my process of finding a solution.	I could do nothing and chalk it up to "a lesson well-learned." or I could go back to the store and explain the situation. or I could write to the manufacturer. or countless other options.

As you will see as you progress through the book, there is another very important reason that your mode of operation becomes Peace. You will soon become very aware of how the thoughts that whirl around in your head occur in a *seemingly* automatic way. They reflect much of who you are and create much of how you are. By regularly (or automatically) coming from a place of Peace, those "automatic" thoughts will also reflect and add to the direction of Peace that you are moving toward. This expedites the process of becoming an effective Peace manager.

What you will also notice over time is that the techniques offered throughout the book not only assist you with choosing Peace (affecting the first tier) but also change your essence, which will, in a sense, influence your second tier.

Peace is a choice! It is that simple! This notion is presented very clearly in *A Course in Miracles.* (p. 90):

I must have decided wrongly, because I am not at peace.
I made the decision myself, but I can also decide otherwise.
I want to decide otherwise, because I want to be at peace.

<u>Exercise (C)</u>:

A Two-Tiered Choice

Goals for this section:

- Become aware that Peace is a choice
- Identify that there are two choices to make when deciding on any words or actions
- When entering a charged situation, choose Peace before you choose any action
- Apply the two-tiered choice to your thoughts

<u>Activity A:</u>

Become acutely aware that you are almost constantly engaged in making decisions about choices of words, choices of actions, and choices or patterns of thoughts.

Put the book down now and go about your normal activities for about ten minutes. Identify how long you go before you are confronted with a thought, needing to speak, or needing to act.

How many choices did you make in that ten minutes?

Are you aware that you were probably not even conscious about what you were thinking, saying, or doing?

Are you aware how you routinely make the decisions to think, speak, or act in a way that is seemingly automatic, haphazard, or simply follows old patterns?

Are you aware that each thought caused a direction (a decision) on how to proceed (even what your next thought would be)?

Now that you are aware of this concept, I will repeat the question:

How many choices did you make in that ten minutes? Countless?

You may have experienced a relatively benign ten minutes, not feeling any charge.

Did you notice if any of your thoughts, words, or actions reflected the spirit or mood you were in, and are you pleased with the choices you made?

If you were stressed, were the choices in line with the way you would like to act?

If you were calm and peaceful, were your patterns of thoughts and choices of words and actions reflecting that state of mind?

Activity B:

Next time you enter a situation that is already charged, take a moment before responding. Make a conscious choice to come from a place of Peace, before you decide which words to say or which action to choose.

Activity C:

The very next person you see, for whatever reason, will be an opportunity to try the two-tiered approach. Say to yourself, "first I choose to come from a place of Peace, then I will proceed in thoughts, words, or actions."

Keep repeating this skill during every opportunity you have.

Activity D:

Next time you are engaged in thought or contemplation about how to handle an upcoming situation, take a time-out. Say to yourself, "this is an opportunity to choose Peace." Then make the choice: "I will come from a place of Peace, not stress or anger." Then go back into your time of thought and contemplation.

Always remember after you try any new technique to spend a moment evaluating it.

5 RELEASE THE DRAMA QUEEN

I realize that as most of you begin reading this, you will think "I can skip over this—it doesn't pertain to me." STOP!! Don't move on just yet. Let me have a moment of your time. This term might not have such a great connotation, but once you see that there is indeed a bit of a Drama Queen in all of us, I believe that you will do what it takes to shake that label.

The "Drama Queen" is the role we play when we engage in conversations or activities that take on a larger significance than the situation warrants. This can be in the amount of time we spend thinking about the situation or the energy that we give to the situation. This amount of attention we give to a situation can be an exaggeration of sorts. This exaggeration should not be something that causes embarrassment. On a subconscious level, this exaggeration actually *represents* something we value. In a very subtle way, at some level, we believe that the drama of life, the exaggerated experience of life, is how we call forth life or life energy.

Most of us would probably agree that we want to experience life to the fullest. For lack of a better way, drama is often our key to "experiencing." What will eventually happen, is that this thing we value, experiencing life to its fullest, will still happen, but it will happen from a place of Peace, not drama or stress.

Our stresses, including emotion-laden relationships and interactions, provide a form of vitality. When we feel this vitality, it may be difficult initially to choose to give up the drama. In fact, I had one student, Cindy, who pulled me aside and very genuinely and bravely told me, "I argue with my mother and shut her out in abrupt ways. We have very heated interactions. I don't want to give this up because it is an outlet for me to explode in a very safe way. I need this now, and it feels good."

This was the first time I was directly presented with the idea that drama felt good. Thankfully, what came to me was a question I posed to her. I asked Cindy, "That good feeling that you experience, how long does it last?" Cindy answered, "while it is happening, and for a few seconds after." She began to see where I was going and her face changed before I even got my next question out. I then asked her "what do you feel after that?" Her eyes gazed at the floor, then back up at me and she said "guilt, sadness and feeling like I tarnish a very important relationship." I followed by saying "Congratulations! You have taken the next step in Peace management, that of 'valuing Peace.' I could not have created a better lesson for you!"

Following that interaction, Cindy became very attentive in the following sessions of the Peace management course. What she learned was that the drama, and its related feeling of exhilaration, is very short lived and not worth the chaos and the negative emotions that it causes.

Since I initially became aware of this possible subconscious desire for drama, it seems to repeatedly come to my attention. Enough so, that I decided to give it special attention in this book. I realize that this has to be dealt with in some people before they are ready to move on and do the work of Peace management.

A friend who sought me out because of a stated desire for Peace management provides an example. At that point she was still not willing to give up the drama and stress to focus on the work of Peace management. I felt as though I was banging my head against the wall. She said she wanted Peace, but she would not stop talking about her multiple stressful situations long enough to even begin discussing the concept of Peace. Unfortunately, I think our time restrictions played a role here. We did all of our work during phone conversations, because when we would meet face to face, her two year old twin daughters had a knack for distracting us from the work at hand. She would call me when her children were napping, and the calls were brief.

Every time my friend and I would begin the work of Peace management, she felt she needed to catch me up on all the stressors in her life. This is where the line between friendship and a professional relationship became blurred. As her friend, she viewed my role as lending a sympathetic ear. It is one I would want to provide for her, because even though I know focusing on stress is a very unhealthy practice, I realize not everyone is immediately ready for Peace and everyone moves along at their own pace. However, the interactions we had scheduled were intended to be time spent on integrating Peace. In my heart, I knew my friend was very attached to the drama because she felt it served her well at that point. I realized working with me would not work for her and she would do better in a group setting or reading the information.

At that point, I decided to acknowledge my friend's stressors and tell her we would pick up Peace management at a time that was better for her. I must say my heart ached, because I knew how much she needed Peace, yet I could see that she viewed the drama, at some level, as necessary for her emotional survival. In the interim, I simply asked her to observe the various stressors, identify the "charge" associated with each, and determine if they were beneficial or detrimental. I believe she already knew the answer. She was taking sleeping pills, an anti-anxiety medication, and an antidepressant. I came to believe that if she were in a group setting, she would not be so focused on her issues and would be able to hear the concepts and strategies. She will be one of the first people who receives a copy of this book.

The major point I would like to make here is that this book is a great format for learning the management process. I cannot hear your stressors. You cannot let them block me from getting the word to you. You can choose to put the book down, but you will not let the magnitude of your stressors block the process. It may be helpful to know that I have seen this program work for people who have experienced stressors that you and I could not even dream of. Yet I must caution you that at various points in this process the Drama Queen may rear her ugly head and distract you from choosing Peace. Confront your stressors, and tell yourself that you will not let them take your attention away from the work at hand.

In the beginning, you will notice that the stressors are all around you, and they eat up a great deal of your time and attention. Peace management does not make the stressors go away. Chaos and drama will continue to exist in the world around you. But you will respond to them differently. After you begin integrating Peace, you will see the stressors as they really are, outside of yourself, simply there to be witnessed and then let go. You will eventually get to a point where you will not even label those outside things as stressors. They will simply exist. But you must take the first step: be willing to take your time, attention, and energy off of the stressors and instead give it to a new way of experiencing all life has to offer.

Do not be too concerned if this part of the process is difficult for you. This difficulty happens to the best of us! A prime example is Kevin, a brilliant hospital administrator. During a business update, Kevin's boss had talked about not having the budget for an additional middle manager or the money for needed project supplies and computers for an upcoming deadline. Kevin responded with a loud and passionate response. His face was red, and he moved his hands in large motions. Later, he seemed to regret his response. After the meeting, I left him my number and asked him to call me.

About one hour after the meeting, Kevin called. He tried to explain his situation. I told him the reason I wanted to talk to him centered around a book I was writing. I introduced the Peace management concept. He seemed interested, but seemed more interested in telling me about his stressors. I asked him if I could meet with him. I felt our conversation needed to be face-to-face. He agreed. He started the face-to-face conversation the same way he began it when we were on the phone, focusing on the stressors and the reason that he had reacted as he did. I was able to intermittently get in the concepts of Peace management. Kevin listened very attentively, but as soon as he would speak he would again refocus on the stressors and their validity.

Well, I went into a different mode. I felt I needed to do my "crash course," which I save for very few people. I believed that with Kevin's schedule, we might never have the opportunity to discuss Peace management again. I started by asking, "are you avoiding the concept of Peace?" He looked at me with a puzzled look. I asked him if he realized that he kept bringing the conversation back to the stressors. He again looked puzzled. I stated, "I don't want to come across as insensitive, but the specific stressors are not my concern. You need to handle them in the way you see fit. They are not my concern or my expertise. What I do care about is your Peace and well-being." I told him I really wanted to work with him, but we could not afford to spend any of our precious time focusing on business management. Well, that was all it took. I left his office 2 ½ hours later, having had the opportunity to delve deeply into Peace management.

I am in no way suggesting that you ignore, repress (to force ideas or impulses that are painful to the conscious mind into the unconscious mind or to prevent unconscious ideas or impulses from reaching the level of consciousness), or suppress (to consciously dismiss from the mind any unacceptable ideas or impulses) the thoughts you have or the emotions you feel. Both of the latter two terms are actually psychiatric terms and represent unhealthy ways of coping. I agree. Your emotions are real. They are the response pattern that has become your habit over your entire life experience. I believe that ignoring and repressing emotions also creates negative consequences. Some professionals might take you down a path of deeply living and experiencing your emotions, in an effort to come out healthy on the other side. I believe if this becomes the mode of operation then we are simply learning to cope and not changing the old, ineffective patterns of experiencing life.

You will not ignore your emotions in this program. As you read in Part I, first you need to identify and label your stressors. You also need to take it one step further and identify the effects, which are felt as a "charge". Once you realize the ill effects on your body as you progress through this program, the stressors take on less significance in your life, therefore decreasing the drama. This allows you to choose how to spend your energy and time more wisely. You will actually learn first hand that the drama is not the way to summon life energy, but actually drains and fatigues you.

On a personal note, I found drama was actually very easy to give up. Once I became aware of the extent of drama in life and how it robbed Peace, I could easily identify drama. I could see how my old self would have handled an issue. I could then see it was a choice to proceed that way or proceed in a different way. It was easy "not to go there." I actually watch other people dwell on their stressors and how they give the stressors a great deal of time or energy. I can identify it as their drama. You can then witness in yourself, and in others, how drama is draining. This recognition makes the choice of "not going there" almost ridiculously easy.

A personal example that demonstrated to me that I was regularly choosing "not to go there" occurred during a phone conversation. One afternoon, I was working in my back yard, enjoying planting flowers. I was in a place of joy. As I answered the phone, almost before I could complete the word "hello," the two people on the other end were screaming at me. I could have easily hung up on them, yelled back, or told them they were fools for acting this way before they had all of the facts. That would have fed into continuing the drama. Without needing to give it much thought, I let them finish their yelling, allowing them to fizzle out on their own.

Then I calmly said, "Why don't you call ___ and find out what really happened. Then we can continue this conversation." I had absolutely zero "charge" and was able to calmly and joyfully return to planting my perennials.

Once you choose to minimize or release the drama, you will experience the feeling of Peace. This could be done simply by asking yourself, "do I want to be a part of the drama?" I can almost guarantee you that the answer will be "no." This will allow you to appreciate the new approach, giving *VALUE* to Peace. Once you see its value, you will be willing to try various strategies that will be presented here. They will allow you to bring Peace to stressful areas of your life and replace previous patterns and habits of behavior.

Exercise (D):

Release the Drama Queen

Goals for this section:

- Identify the areas of your life which create the biggest "charge" in your body
- Honestly confront the charge areas to determine if they take on a bigger charge or significance than you feel the situation realistically warrants (and the key here is honesty)
- Separate the time that you think or talk about your stressors from the time you spend working on Peace management, gradually reducing the former activity

---

Activity A:

List the areas that currently create the biggest "charge" for you:

1. ________________________________

2. ________________________________

3. ________________________________

4. ________________________________

5. ________________________________

6. ________________________________

List the areas that you would currently identify as your "buttons" and identify those who push them:

1. ________________________________

2. ________________________________

3. ________________________________

4. ________________________________

5. ________________________________

6. ________________________________

Now go back to your lists and identify if there are any (at least one area) that could be considered your "drama" (one that takes on a bigger charge or significance than you feel the situation realistically warrants—possibly an exaggerated response)

Now go back and evaluate that list one more time. *Honesty is the key*. You don't have to answer to anyone but yourself. There is no need to prove anything to anyone, and there is no need to maintain pride. You are by yourself. If you do not begin by being honest with yourself, you will eventually come to a block in this program. We all have to swallow our pride, realizing that it truly is more important to be at Peace than it is to be right. In the big picture, it really doesn't matter if you are right or not. Think of the book title *Don't Sweat the Small Stuff, and it's* ***All*** *Small Stuff* by Richard Carlson. This certainly puts things in perspective.

Activity B:

If you are finding that you are having trouble letting go of your drama or thoughts about your stressors, journaling might be necessary. Journaling is almost like writing in a diary. It is information that only you will use. It is an outlet and an opportunity for growth. In this case, it is writing down events or situations and your reflections on these situations. This will be a way to compartmentalize your thoughts.

- allow time for journaling and reflecting on your stressors—the magnitude, the significance, and the consequences.
- When you are not journaling, train your mind to let your stressors fade from your mind. If you find you are unable to do this and are giving stressors attention again - time to go back to the journal. Allow that time to be the only time you contemplate these stressors.
- Work on your current strategy of Peace management throughout the rest of the day.

Note: an alternative to journaling is identifying one location that will be used for you to think about your stressors. An example might be a rocking chair upstairs. I frequently advise this strategy when someone is going through a divorce. A divorce affects so many facets of one's life and can creep into one's thoughts at very unusual times. I ask the individual to either go immediately to the place they have chosen, or if it is impossible to get there at that time, to make a mental note, so that the thoughts can be dealt with later. Immediately go back to Peace. The time in that chair should be the *only time* you allow yourself to deal with stressors. Otherwise, stressful matters rob your Peace on a continual basis. Please realize this strategy is not the mainstay of Peace management. It is actually a form of stress management. However, in an attempt to gradually minimize the Drama Queen and the effect it has of robbing your Peace, it is one of the early techniques for working in the direction of Peace.

DEVELOP TRUE POWER

6

If there is anything that will help you value Peace, it is understanding that coming from a place of Peace is the only way to experience true power. This is especially critical in attempting to replace anger with Peace. Often people feel angry when they feel powerless, out of control, or feel a sense of hopelessness or helplessness.

In an attempt to feel in control of a situation or in control of themselves, people will occasionally exert an external control. External control means having control over someone or something else. This creates a sense of power. However, that is an erroneous thought, as it is not true power at all, but rather a form of manipulation.

When someone forces their control over another, the "victim" responds by succumbing as a means of avoiding further confrontation. It is a surrender of sorts. It is a passive action, possibly rooted in fear. Therefore, the one exerting control over the other does not actually earn power. It merely *appears* as if the controlling individual has power. There is no true satisfaction or feeling of joy in using this type of manipulation.

True power is a benefit that develops naturally as you become a better Peace manager. True power is accompanied by a feeling of joy, satisfaction, and Peace. Peace brings it on, and Peace is the result. It is cyclic.

As indicated, although power is a benefit of Peace, there will be instances when the desire to feel true power becomes the driving force as you develop a plan for a situation. This became very clear to me when I went to pick up my son from a dance.

My best friend and I arrived at the school twenty minutes early to pick up the boys. I went up to the door to see if our boys were ready to leave. They were nowhere in sight, so I sat on the curb near the door. A ruckus broke out, and it drew my attention and interest. There was a young girl, probably around thirteen years old, who was out of control. This was obviously a continuation of a problem that had begun earlier, as the two adult chaperones at the door were not surprised at her behavior and seemed to know about the situation. I couldn't hear exactly what was being said initially, but the girl was crying, screaming, and hitting her head against an outside brick wall.

The girl wanted to leave and walk home, but the adults would not let her leave early without a parent there for pick-up. She kept trying to convince them and started screaming about an altercation she had had with another girl. After the girl re-entered the building, I talked to the woman at the door. The woman identified herself as a juvenile case worker and said "she is one of our emotionally troubled teens." My heart ached for the girl and her inability to cope and have Peace.

When the teen returned she was still screaming and crying. I briefly told the woman and man (a father chaperone) at the door about my book and asked if they would allow me to speak to the teen for about 30 seconds, presuming she is willing. The woman at the door agreed to let me ask the girl's permission to talk to her. The woman was soon off with another child who was sick and needed a phone. I asked the girl if I could talk to her for a minute. I told her I was a nurse and thought I could help her. She agreed to listen.

The girl's name was Kathy. I knew I only had her for a brief period of time, so my window of opportunity to help this girl was very small. I focused on what I perceived was the main issue. That was power and control. I told her that her anger and sadness really made my heart ache. I could sense that she was feeling powerless and out of control. She agreed. I told her that the other girl, named Lindsey had robbed her Peace. I told Kathy that she was the only one who could give permission to give her Peace away.

I assured Kathy she would feel powerful and Peace-full if she took charge of herself and didn't let the other girl, or any situation, take away her Peace. She was in charge of it. I challenged her to give this a try. I asked her to remain at the door and keep her Peace, no matter whom she interacted with or who tried to agitate her and rob her Peace. I assured her I would remain outside the door if she needed a little coaching or support. She agreed.

After a few minutes, Lindsey returned to the door. Kathy looked over her shoulder at me, tipped her head and pointed with her eyes, letting me know that this girl had been her nemesis. I winked at her and she smiled. I was extremely proud of this young woman. She remained composed and calm during the entire interaction with Lindsey. The father at the door was amazed. His jaw was at his navel the entire time. He asked what I had done. As I saw my son leaving the building, more than ready to go home, I just said "buy the book, this story will definitely be in there." So, chaperone father . . . now you know what happened. I helped Kathy understand how to experience her true power.

The calm, joy, and satisfaction Kathy felt was a direct result of her ability to protect her Peace. And this might have been the first time she experienced Peace and the true power that accompanies it. She felt authentic power. That is inner power, achieved by choosing Peace as the place you live life, experience moments, and interact with others.

The power that results from Peace is such a healthy power. It feels so right. It is nothing like the false power experienced when it is forced over others or comes from a particular position you hold, as in a job or as a parent. I have the feeling of being in control when I choose to come from a place of Peace during an interaction. I might sense that I am going to enter an interaction that would normally bring on a charge. I go into it knowing that this is an opportunity to practice Peace. And that is exactly what I do.

I must say, this approach often fosters a good resolution, but that is not the issue. Because even if the results of the interaction aren't as I hoped, I still come away feeling the inner power for choosing Peace and not diverting from it.

I feel so strongly about this issue that it is the driving force leading me to another book and program. My hope is that this specialized version of the Peace management program will be adopted by the court system to replace the currently mandated anger management courses. I am joining forces with experts in the field to create an effective program for some of the people who need it most: those who manifest their anger in such an extreme way that they actually break the law.

True power comes from the self control we feel as we choose Peace. We know the benefits: physical health, emotional stability, authentic power, and the resulting Peace.

7
Immediate Peace/Immediate Relief

If there is anything that will convince you that a Peace management program is "worth it", it will be the first time you successfully incorporate Peace management in a real life encounter and feel immediate relief. This will provide a jump start to set you on your way to valuing Peace, followed by a willingness to implement the various strategies. I have a wonderful example to share with you:

> I was working the 3-11 shift the day after Christmas. We were very short staffed. Needless to say, it was very busy and the patients, unfortunately, got little more than basic care that evening. In fact, I had just called my husband to tell him not to expect me home on time.
>
> As I was quickly walking down the hall with a chart, trying to catch a physician before he left the division, I noticed a patient who was a rather distinguished gentleman of middle eastern descent, standing sideways against his door. He had a very tense look on his face and had obviously been crying. I stopped

dead in my tracks. He was not my patient, I did not have any report on him, yet at first glance I sensed he was in desperate need of medical attention and Peace management. I didn't know his problems or issues, but I started asking questions quickly to try to get him some assistance. He was beyond what we call frustrated, and his pain was multi-tiered. The immediate issue was chest pain and anxiety. I helped him return to bed, placed him on oxygen, and called for his nurse. I gave him a brief discussion on how his anxiety was aggravating his chest pain and causing his heart to receive less blood and oxygen during this period of need. I promised him I would not leave his room until I knew that he had the help he needed. I also told him that he needed to take my next directions seriously and "trust me on this one."

I didn't have time to do a Peace management crash course; I needed results NOW! I went directly to the core. I said "I promise I will get you all the medical and health interventions you need to correct the underlying problem, but you need to trust me on this first step. We need to get rid of this anxiety and stress before it does you real damage." He agreed in that moment. I said "it is really easy, but it has to come from the depths of you." He understood. I said "Okay. Right now you need to choose Peace." He gave me a half smile and said "are you serious?" I responded "you have no idea how serious I am. You *have to* choose Peace." He took a deep breath, closed his eyes for about ten seconds, opened his eyes, and smiled at me. He didn't need to say a word to me, because I was aware of what had taken place. He knew that I knew what happened, but he wanted to give me the word of confirmation. He said "the chest pain is gone, and I know I am going to be okay". The intern soon came in and began the battery of tests.

> Later that evening, the man and I had a brief conversation. He let me in on his history and stressors. He was a long term diabetic with a cardiac history. He was fifty nine years old and had an eight month old at home with a "much younger wife." She was currently in another hospital being treated for a severe, debilitating neuromuscular disorder. This man needed the full program!

The choice for Peace, in order to achieve immediate relief, does not need to be related to improving your physical health in the moment. Just think back to that troubled teen, Kathy. She chose Peace and it dramatically affected her emotional well-being in a flash. She experienced the rewards in an instant.

Another wonderful example is described in the written words of one of my nursing students, Diana. She turned in this story as part of one of her assignments. She has allowed me to include it, with only some minor editing, because she wanted to share what she and her son experienced. Diana is very in touch with her own spirituality, and she calls upon it as a way to bring her Peace. Here is Diana's story:

> My ten year old son and I were riding in the car together to go to a function. My son was still angry at something his cousin had done to make him mad. The more my son thought about it, the more agitated and angry he became. I was trying to stop the escalation of anger by gently hinting that he should let it go. This made him angrier, and I was feeling negative energy radiating from this small boy. His negativity was so powerful that it began affecting my energy. I could feel the instant change in my body and my thought process. My heart was breaking for my son, who has been through so much in his young life: a divorce, a dad who is ill, three moves and three schools in the last one and a half years, a mom who has to work, a mom who has gone back to

school. How could he even begin to see the light at the end of the tunnel?!

Finally, my son's emotions were so out of control that he just broke down and sobbed. You know, the heart-wrenching "I've had enough and I can't take any more" cry. I was so laden with guilt and powerlessness. I was at a loss about what to do. This is when God came to my rescue. The next words out of my mouth were not mine. I can only say I believe He put them there. I said "Michael, all this stuff inside us, that is hurting us, is too big for us to handle alone. Let's ask God to help us by taking all these thoughts and anger away because God is powerful enough to help us with them. Let's be quiet and ask God to help us and tell him that we really need his love today."

We were silent, each in our own little prayer. Not ten minutes later, Michael turned to me with one of those lighten-a-mom's-heart smiles. "Mom look, there's a rainbow on me!" I looked, and sure enough there was a rainbow on him. Giggling, he said, "I guess that makes me the pot of gold." I gave him a smile and silently I said "it sure does!", thanking God. We're gonna make it!

WHAT A STORY!!!

I have experienced situations like this in my own life, and I have also been able to coach others into choosing Peace during the heat of the battle. I truly value Peace all of the time, but it is most obvious when I experience immediate relief.

Exercise (E):

Immediate Peace / Immediate Relief

Goal for this section:

- Choose Peace during an intense period of stress or anger

Activity:

This exercise will just be presented here. There is no immediate work, as it needs to be implemented during the heat of the moment.

Just give this thought some attention now. Imagine using it during a stressful moment.

Next time you are experiencing an intensely stressful moment, stop in your tracks. From the depths of your being, say "I choose Peace NOW!!!!!"

Close your eyes (unless of course you are driving or operating heavy machinery).

When you open your eyes, revel in the marvelous results.

Part 3:

Techniques

SIMPLE, NOT EASY

8

As you begin this section of techniques, realize you actually have already begun implementing some techniques in the section on Valuing and Protecting. However, now is the time when you will most likely feel you are doing the "work" of the program.

I would like you to realize this work will be simple, not easy. Sound confusing? Actually the words represent very different concepts. "Simple" means that it is not complicated and has one feature. What you will see is that all the techniques have a common goal related to one concept. That is to *assist you* with *choosing* Peace. Actually, Peace management is so simple that instead of a book there could have been a pamphlet that had only two words in it: "choose Peace." The various techniques give you different approaches to assist you with working Peace into various situations in your life. Some techniques will resonate with you. Some will not.

"Easy" means not difficult. Although the process of Peace management is simple, it can be very difficult. The difficulty comes into play because Peace management requires a change. Change is not something that most of us embrace. In fact, most people resist change. That is why it was so important to introduce this concept slowly, allowing you to get a taste of Peace. This slow transition allows you the opportunity to experience the value of it, and provides the impetus to pursue learning the techniques that will bring about the ultimate change to successful Peace management. A change in behavior requires repeated reinforcement. That is the purpose of my intention that Peace management is implemented as a twenty week course.

As previously mentioned, we have a vested interest in doing things "the way we have always done them." Habits provide a sense of comfort and stability. You now need to be willing to change your entire essence. A pretty scary thought!! But I and many others can testify that "it was all worth it, that we like ourselves and life much better, and we are never going back."

I am not being naïve when I say Peace management can actually be easy, especially when the desire for Peace is strong. My career and life encounters allow me exposure to people with extreme life situations, more extreme and numerous than most people will ever experience. I have watched many lives transform after exposure to Peace management. Hopefully, after going through the whole program, you will join in my sentiment that Peace management is not only simple but also very easy. If you do not share that sentiment, I hope you will at least agree that Peace management is definitely worth the effort.

If you experience periods of difficulty or internal resistance (coming from something within yourself), take a break. Identify the blocks, analyze them, reestablish a plan, and get yourself back on track. If you experience any external resistance (coming from something outside of yourself—someone else or a situation), my recommendation is: *don't let that stop you.* You need to be ruthlessly selfish in this endeavor. The change you experience may scare others. It will most likely result from the fear of how it might impact on your relationship with them. Explain that Peace management will certainly benefit them and your relationship in the long run. Simply ask for their blessing and patience.

As we begin the actual techniques, you will notice that they fall in one of four categories. However, there are only a few that purely fall into one clean, nicely labeled category. There is an overlap in most techniques, and learning Peace management is a general process, rather than a linear progression.

The four categories of the techniques that are included are:

1. maintaining Peace in a known or expected stressful situation
2. promoting stillness or quieting of the mind
3. removing or reducing the toxicity (or blocks) to Peace
4. promoting a new way of being

There is no specific order that is used, but it may be helpful to follow in the order I have laid out, as occasionally my terminology builds on a previously mentioned concept. However, if you are intrigued by a certain topic or title because it applies to what is currently going on in your life, jump to it. Just realize it may not be as clear or easy to grasp as it would be if you had already worked through some of the building blocks.

The first several techniques are fairly concrete and easy to grasp and apply when you are a new Peace manager. The later techniques assume you have a basic understanding of the program, and concepts are more abstract. The more abstract concepts are intended to take you to a higher level of Peace management. Some of the more abstract concepts also allow you to remove the blocks that keep you from experiencing life from a place of Peace on a regular basis.

In the beginning of my development as a Peace manager, I used the techniques often and in a way that seemed mechanical. It was simply part of the process for me. I can now say that I am approaching the point where it really is the "way that I am." I don't even need the techniques or my "mechanical-feeling" reminders. Peace management is very natural. This process will probably take most of you much less time than it took me, because it was not a clearly defined program for me. There are now clear exercises and goals for each component of this program.

The main goal of the Peace manager is to live every moment and experience every experience from a place of Peace. The *management* idea comes in at various levels. The core of Peace management is *choosing* Peace in every moment. It is that simple! As a manager of Peace, you are making that choice.

However, there is more to it when you look at Peace management as a total way of living. You, as a manager, must also set yourself up to experience Peace so that it happens more often and more automatically. You do this by utilizing appropriate techniques that work for you at different times. The choice of techniques will depend on the situation, your current progress as a manager, and the circumstances. Practicing these techniques will gradually move you toward being a very effective Peace manager.

There are several techniques presented. One pitfall that my full-day seminar participants meet is that they try to fit all their problems into the two or three techniques on which their particular small group is working. Don't try to fit a round peg into a square hole and don't try to fit a square peg into a round hole. Just find all the appropriate square holes and round holes. And if you can't find one that fits perfectly, go get a drill.

You will notice that as you progress, the techniques actually become more gentle and Peaceful themselves. For example, in the beginning you might have to use some of what I call the harsher techniques, such as Removing Toxicity or the Academy Award Winner. But as you become a more skilled manager, the techniques that you seem to pick become more gentle, until you get to a point where you don't even consciously use techniques. Peace-full is just the way you are.

This program can be applied by anyone from any background. I am not aware of any philosophy or religion that would oppose the idea of people managing their Peace. You are simply learning how to find your Peace and then protecting it, which is managing it. One friend who is a fundamentalist Christian admitted that in the beginning, not having read the book, but only having heard a few concepts, she did not like the term Peace management. She felt Peace management meant managing God. That was a real eye opener for me, as my intention has never been to manage God. I could never accomplish that, nor if it were possible, even want to consider it! How I ended up explaining this to my friend, knowing she was very religious, was to tell her that "if she would like to use the literal translation, she could think of it as managing the way she lets God manifest in her life, and that He can manifest as Peace."

In a nutshell, the concept of *managing* your Peace is the guiding of your travels from a place of being absorbed by and responsive to stress and anger, to a place of Peace.

There are many wonderful sacred, spiritual, and religious texts which teach paths for attaining Peace. They are very helpful to countless people. However, occasionally, the wording holds me up. I get stuck on trying to figure out the meaning of the complex verbiage. I get hung up to the point where I focus so much time trying to figure out what is meant that it leaves little time and energy for applying the concepts so that I can experience Peace. And experiencing Peace is what it is all about. It is often said, "knowing about something is the boobie prize." Boy do I get that! I would rather *experience* Peace than *know* every detail about it.

The program of Peace management functions at the level of the ego, with hopes that people will be started on a path which will allow deeper inquiry. That means that this program tries to assist you, *as a person* who is trying to function and remain healthy is this chaotic world. There are many other programs that try to assist you with functioning at a deeper level. I often felt lacking in this ability when working through other programs, because my ego (my person) was trying to figure out things that are beyond the ego. I still have interest in these philosophies for the academic stimulation and assistance on my journey. Yet I know my ego will never grasp these concepts completely. Peace management is something my ego understands.

My hope for people on a more advanced path is that they continue on that path which is beneficial to them, while simultaneously working in this program to improve their health and every day maintenance of Peace. You may notice some similarities in the various programs, yet Peace management allows identification with the ego.

I would like to remind you . . . it could be as simple as a choice in any given moment.

You will probably develop your own techniques as you go along. I would love to hear what works for you. In fact, many of my students have been willing to share their own creations. With their permission, I have included some of them in this book. This sharing of techniques is actually my hope for people who start up Peace management study groups. The section for groups and group facilitators that is presented in this book will guide groups who see the advantage of utilizing feedback, tips, and techniques from others going through the process.

I trust you will discover that any work you put forth in becoming a Peace manager will be well rewarded. Once you reap the benefits, you will be able to identify with the story below:

> There were two dragonfly larvae at the bottom of the pond. They spent many months together maturing and changing. They noticed a strange phenomenon. Every so often, one of the other larvae would float to the top of the water. Once they reached the top, they would leave and never come back. The two larvae found this a very curious occurrence. They discussed it, but could not figure it out. One of the larvae said "I will go to the

> top, leave, check it out, then come back and tell you about it." Off he went. He made it to the top. As he reached the surface, his skin split and molted. He had wings! He flew away. You guessed it . . . he never went back. There are two reasons for this: once you have your wings you can't go back, and once you have your wings you don't want to go back.

Embrace the change, enjoy the journey, and see if others want to travel on this path with you. I speak from experience when I tell you that once you "get it" you want to take everyone along with you.

Technique: Self Talk

I chose to start with this technique because it is very easy, can be applied to most situations, and works so well for me and others. And as the cliché goes:

This is not Rocket Science!!

Self Talk is incredibly easy, almost to the point where you will chuckle at how simple and effective it is. Your reaction to a situation changes the moment you engage in self talk. I have one student who hits his forehead with the heel of his hand every time he realizes the he has not engaged in self talk. He knows Self Talk works for him immediately.

"Self talk" is identifying what is making you stressed or angry, then simply saying

"is stress or anger going to make the situation better (or go away)?"

The answer is always "no." Then the next part is reinforcing the effect and saying to yourself

"the only consequence of my stress or anger is that it will harm me."

When you are actually using self talk for your situation, you will be more specific in your words. Situation specific language drives the need home faster and harder. *For example:* next time you are in traffic and running behind schedule, simply say to yourself "is my stress going to get me there faster? My stress will only hurt me and not help the situation." Now, being a skilled driver or catching a break with lane changes might get you there faster, but the stress will not affect the clock.

Recently, I thought someone very close to me had diabetes. I am well aware of the course and consequences of this disease. A normal reaction would be to feel stress about the possibility. Luckily, I was already very successful at Peace management. I simply used the self talk technique. It went something like this:

> Okay - if he has diabetes, my stress is *not* going to make it go away. And if he does have diabetes and I am stressed, he will pick up on it and he will become stressed. If it is diabetes and he is stressed, that will raise his blood sugar. His first medical encounter will be a crisis. This will probably leave him with fear of the disease. My stress has no purpose and function in this situation. It can only bring harm to him and me!

I truly did not experience stress or any other negative emotion during the entire situation.

Sharing another personal example, I was in Mexico with my husband. My son was back home, playing baseball. He was hit in the head with a baseball. I was told "it shattered his skull and he had a brain injury." Now, just a side note: he actually had a head injury, which is very different than a brain injury. Nonetheless, that is what I was told. I was told he had a blood clot in his head and learned he had to have surgery to drain the clot and have a metal plate placed to support his skull. I don't think any skill with Peace management could have helped in that initial moment when I learned of his injury. I felt as though I had lost all circulation from my body and that I was about to pass out. But something came to me quickly, and that was self talk. I said to myself:

> Stress is not going to turn back the clock and make him wear the helmet during warm up. It is not going to change the outcome of the surgery or recovery. I need to put a lot of things in motion here to get information and get home as quickly as possible. My

stress will only block my clear thinking (which I need right now) and it will only harm me.

Well, I must say, this attitude and technique worked for me. My husband noted that I was incredibly calm and level headed as I tried to find an English speaking operator at 10:30 p.m. In fact, we needed to go out to another hotel because only Spanish speaking people were working the night shift at our hotel. We found out that the airport closes at night (locked doors, lights off, no employees). This is not something that most of us have been confronted with. The next plane out was 3:30 the next afternoon. I had to maintain my Peace that entire time. Without Peace management techniques, I don't know how I would have succeeded. I must say, I probably only slept a little over one hour that night, but I had absolutely zero charge during the entire time.

You can also help others with Self Talk. Sometimes, when others are in a charged situation, they forget that Peace management is appropriate or called for. However, from the outside, it is very clear to us. Sometimes a gentle reminder is all that is needed. Possibly a joke or a brief instruction suggesting specific Self Talk would be helpful.

Obviously, my husband lives with me. He has a built in Peace management advisor. A situation that occurred recently touches on this in a comical sort of way.

On an icy cold January day (the thermometer registered 3°F), Gary came up to the office, held out his empty hand and said "here is the $200 from Tom." Mr. Calm (my nickname for Gary, because he is one of the few people I know who really innately and in an unlearned fashion lives Peace 99% of the time) had a red face, though his color could have been from the arctic temperature, his mannerisms were out of character. I knew he had a charge because I knew all he had done to promote the sale of one of his cars.

- Gary initially showed the car for the first time to Tom on a day when it was 7° F.

- The car was parked behind another undriven car and both were covered with about 18" of snow.
- Gary was late coming home due to the road conditions, but Tom was on time, so Tom stood and watched while Gary labored to clean off both cars.
- The car needed to be jumped, as the battery was low.
- A suggestion that Tom come back on another night went unanswered.
- After the car was started, dug out of the snow, and warmed up, Tom took it for a ride. He liked it but wanted to see the body free of snow, so Gary used warm water to remove the remaining snow and ice from the entire car.
- Gary negotiated a lower price with Tom because Tom was so patient. Tom said he would return in two days with a $200 deposit.
- Tom stayed for 3 hours.
- Tom came back a second time to give Gary the deposit. Gary was not home. The car doors were frozen closed due to the water having been run over the car two nights previously. Tom pulled so hard on the door handles that he shortened the rod that activates the door latch. Tom didn't want to leave a deposit until the car doors were fixed. Gary had to remove both door panels in similarly cold weather and repair them.
- Tom came back today with his wife to buy the car. She didn't like it. Gary was less than happy.

This is where I come in again. I did my wifely duty. I asked, "Do you have a charge?" Gary responded, "A little." I then said "Is your stress going to sell the car to Tom?" He looked at me with that silly grin he now gives me when I engage him in this exercise. He said, "It's actually anger and … okay, it's gone." Then we talked about the sequence of ridiculous events and the set of frustrating factors. Gary was able to talk about the situation from his baseline of Peace.

This is a clear example of the benefit of this program when more than one person in a household or close friends are Peace managers. You help each other come to baseline quickly when there are breaks in being the Gatekeeper in the first place. And we all have our slip-ups.

I also regularly counsel many of my nursing students about the use of "self talk." As they are nursing *students*, they are not always proficient or efficient in the way they perform their work. This often sets them up for stress, disappointment with themselves, or fear. Therefore, in situations that typically cause stress, the first words out of my mouth are, "stress is not going to make this go easier." I ask my students to choose Peace, then support them and assure them that the tasks ahead will go more smoothly if they stay in that place. This approach serves us well. If my students stay in that place of Peace, all goes much better—for all of us!

You will now have the opportunity to try self talk to maintain your Peace. Remember to evaluate this technique, as well as each technique, as you try them. These techniques will become a sound repertoire for you to call on to prevent stress or other negative emotions.

Exercise (F):

Self Talk

Goals for this section:

- Identify areas that are currently causing you stress or anger
- Create the self talk wording that can be used in these specific situations
- Begin utilizing this practice throughout the day

Activity A:

List the areas of your life that are currently causing you stress or anger:

1. (A) example: *I lose my keys at least once a week* ________

2. (A) ____

3. (A) ____

4. (A) ____

5. (A) ____

Now write out the self talk sentence that corresponds with each of the above situations (remember to be specific and also follow up with "it will only hurt me":

1. (B) example: *Stress will not help me find my keys. It will only hurt me.*

2. (B) ____

____

3. (B) ____

____

4. (B) ____

____

5. (B) ____

____

Activity B:

Make a conscious effort to try this out several times during the next few days, until you are doing it automatically.

Evaluate how this technique works for you:

Technique: Change the Thought

This technique is the foundation for Peace management. The rest of the program is built upon this concept. The goal for this program is to go through life experiences without a "charge" in the body. The "charge" is the way you know you are experiencing the release of chemicals, triggered by a negative emotion. Said differently, the goal is to be able to function amidst stressful life circumstances and maintain Peace. If you experience the "charge" that you identified in the first exercise of this book, your body is experiencing the stress. If you are experiencing the stress, you are hurting your body.

Remember, you can not, at will, go directly into your body and turn off the Autonomic Nervous System (ANS). It doesn't work that way. Maybe an easier illustration would be the flip side of this concept. You cannot sit in your chair and say "I am going to feel angry" or "I am going to feel stress." You cannot create a charge on command. Now, you can think of something that makes you angry or stressed, then experience the charge. But you simply cannot do it without the generating thought.

Okay, now let's try this in relation to Peace management. You cannot have a thought that causes you stress and then say, "I am not going to let it affect my Autonomic Nervous System". Sorry, the ANS is on "auto pilot." Remember, you don't have control of the ANS. Your control lies in the choice for Peace. This control and choice occur on two levels. One level is immediate and the other level is the gradual process of becoming a consistent Peace manager.

The immediate technique to employ in order to avoid the response of the ANS is to change the thought. You will be given a few exercises in the next few sections to learn how to do this. The second level just happens automatically as you get further into the program and become a better Peace manager.

How do I change the thought? This is where the real work begins. At this point, I will only be introducing the thought changing process and allowing you to witness how your thought causes the emotional response. You will be introduced to many techniques and exercises to learn to change the thought in order to eliminate the negative emotional response.

All that is asked at this point is that you become aware that the thought (and its meaning to you or your perception) is what causes the negative emotion. I use an exercise with my students to drive home the point that it is the meaning of their thought that creates the stress. There is nothing inherently stressful in the word or concept. I hold up a card for my students that has these letters on it:

maxe lanif

I then ask them if they are experiencing any charge in their body. I usually get a unanimous "no," but sometimes a student will say "yes" because they know that they are being set up for a demonstration, and they experience a bit of anxiety. Yet, nonetheless, the overwhelming answer is "no." I then hold up another card that has the letters spelled out in reverse. The card now reads "final exam." Well, you guessed it. Now I get an overwhelming "yes" when I ask my students if they are experiencing a charge. It is simply their thought about the word or the meaning they give to it, not the letters or the word the letters make up.

In this next exercise, you will begin using what I call "charge cards." There is no intention to get a charge out of you simply by the name of the cards. But I do realize that the word "charge cards," also known as "credit cards" will create a charge in some of you. This exercise will give you an opportunity to examine what causes a charge for you. The words on your charge cards will be used at various points throughout this program. The only goal of the cards in this initial introduction of them is to identify that there are concepts that create a charge for you. You will also have the opportunity to individualize your deck for later use.

Exercise (G):

Change the Thought

Goals for this section:

- Continue to identify areas that are currently causing you stress or anger
- Become aware that your thought about something (the generating thought) is what causes the emotion or charge
- Individualize the charge card deck and begin utilizing self talk or any other technique you create at this point to minimize the charge you feel when looking at the words you identified as provoking a stress response

Activity A:

Either cut out the individual charge cards at the end of this exercise section or make your own on 3x5 cards. Also, cut out several blank cards. Turn the cards face down. Turn them over one at a time and watch your reaction to the words. Make a pile of the cards that are your "provocative words." These are the words that provoke or create a charge in your body. They represent the generating thought.

Take the blank cards and write down words that were not in this deck that are individualized sources of charge for you. An example would be something like "moving" or "being fired." These words are not in the deck, but they may have special meaning for you and create a charge.

Activity B:

Begin practicing with these cards. It is a very safe and non-confrontational way to begin identifying the specific things (or generating thoughts) that routinely give you a charge.

Start playing with this idea. You know about the technique of self talk. You can try self talk with your charge cards. The eventual goal of this exercise is for you to go through the entire deck and have no charge.

Try any other technique you can think of to begin minimizing the effect each word has on you. As you learn more techniques in this program, pull out these cards again and try the new techniques. You will get to the point where nothing (on paper at least) will provoke a charge. It is the start of application to real life.

deadline	traffic jam
IRS	defiant children
mother-in-law	boss

mother	father
April 15th	being late
piled-up laundry	parents

paying bills	neighbors
doctor appointments	health problems
ex-husband	ex-wife

criticism

hostile people

late to work

price of gas

brother

sister

lawyer	homework
death	back to school
the holidays	traffic cop

judge	car repairs
car break-down	child abuse
domestic violence	loss

animal abuse	war
impotence	weight gain
sex	home maintenance

electrical storm

elevators

back home

driving in snow

telemarketer

behind schedule

debt	mortgage
heights	kid's schedule
relatives	mornings

bedtime	divorce
break-up	poor drivers
blind date	fixed income

Technique: It's Your Choice

This technique follows nicely after "Change the Thought." As noted earlier, Peace management views Peace as a choice, in all but a few instances. The choice centers on choosing Peace by changing the thought. As you can see, these two techniques are very intermingled. They are separated solely for the purpose of presentation. This separation is done to make it easier to grasp the process. It is a new skill you are learning. It helps to understand what all of the components are as you try to put it together to work for you.

Early in your practice, the choice may feel very mechanical or artificial. This occurs because you are taking time out to make a conscious choice. Later the choice will still be conscious, but it will occur at a very different level. It will still be conscious, because it will still be a part of your awareness. However, there will be no time allotted to this step. Peace just takes the driver's seat. In the beginning, you will essentially take a moment to say to yourself "I choose Peace," then you will begin your interaction or action. Eventually, Peace will become so comfortable to you that it will simply be the way you operate. It will almost be as if there isn't even another option. You will have integrated it into your being. This will be you!

This transformation can happen rather quickly for some. My nursing students are in my nursing course for five weeks. They receive a condensed course in Peace management while they are with me. I ask them do a great deal of work during that five weeks and ask for a lot of feedback, in an effort to keep refining the program. Some students move through very quickly. Some of the comments I receive are like this: "I have a long way to go, yet I am already a different person, choosing Peace without needing to give it much thought. I like how this feels."

In most situations that you will deal with, there will be a choice. I choose to come from a place of Peace, or I choose to let stress/anger be my mode of operation. Occasionally, there will not be a choice. In those instances, you will have what is known as a primitive response. Essentially, instinct takes over. But these will actually be the rare occasions.

Your body was designed to appropriately respond to a threat of physical danger. It assists with physical survival. What I am referring to is what is commonly called the "fight or flight response." If you were a cave man or lived in a jungle with ferocious animals, the fight or flight response would serve you well. Your body is equipped to quickly release chemicals that could make you fight the lion or run like heck. However, most of you live in buildings and have poodles or kitties in your living area. It is quite ridiculous for us to utilize such a powerful response in dealing with our bosses, our mates, the clerks at the mall, or anyone else who elicits a powerful response from us. Not all our situations match the level of the response needed when meeting a lion face-to-face. Yet the response to lower level stressors creates gradual wear and tear on your body.

When imminent danger is present, or even the possibility of physical danger is there, your body responds appropriately. I would never suggest attempting Peace management in these circumstances. Your body is responding in a way that gives you the tools you need to attempt to effectively handle the situation. It is a good thing to feel the charge in these situations.

Examples might help you to understand when the fight or flight response could come into play for you. If you were swimming in a river and suddenly found yourself being pulled away quickly, needing possibly to swim against a current, the stress response would kick in. This would bring all your strength, speed, and power to you in the moment. It would provide you the best opportunity possible to struggle for your survival. Peace management would not serve you well in this situation.

Another example that might initiate a functional (or helpful and appropriate) stress response would be in response to a loud noise. Loud or unexpected noises initiate a fear which triggers this response in your body. I just experienced a great example of this. This example will also demonstrate how I can allow the stress response to be there when needed, but quickly differentiate and not allow nonfunctional stress to enter the picture.

I was carrying a large basket through the kitchen and met resistance. I obviously knocked something over, because there was an immediate loud noise. The functional stress response allowed me to move out of the way quickly and avoid being hurt by the crashing objects. This was the "flight" effect of the "fight or flight response." This is something your body automatically does for you. The next part of the story demonstrates how Peace management worked for me. It "kicked in" without me even making it a deliberate step. And this all happened in the span of about two seconds. I looked at what had been broken. It was several pieces of tableware that have sentimental value to me. Even though they were irreplaceable, I did not experience any charge for their loss.

In my former way of living, losing these items would have stressed me, creating a definite charge. In fact, when similar things like this had happened in the past, I would not have been able to clean up the mess in that moment. I would have been too charged. I would need to clean up later or have someone else do it, so that I did not resurrect the charge. Now it almost seems ridiculous to me that I would ever have allowed a charge in my body, tearing down my health in the process, for something that now seems so silly and cannot be reversed by the charge. I am very aware of the loss, but choose not to experience stress over it.

And like I said, I did not even say "I choose Peace" when I looked at the mess. It just is the way that I am. As I was just starting to use this technique, I would have needed that brief moment to back away and say "I choose Peace" before I would have let myself identify what I broke.

Initially, you may grow tired of reading "choose Peace," but it is the core of the program. As you move through the process you will begin to say it over and over again yourself. It will be a mantra, of sorts. Eventually, you will move to a new level where you do not even have to make an overt effort of choosing Peace. It will be automatic, the way you live.

Peace really is your choice, whether it happens by taking the moment to say or think "I choose Peace," or it is the result of the underlying choice that you made to start the Peace management process which changed the way you now act automatically. I made the choice for Peace. I will never choose otherwise!

Again, I would like to cite the quote from A Course in Miracles:

I must have decided wrongly, because I am not at peace.
I made the decision myself, but I can also decide otherwise.
I want to decide otherwise, because I want to be at peace.

Exercise (H):

It's Your Choice

Goal for this section:

- Practice making Peace a conscious choice

Activity:

Over the next few days, say to yourself (or out loud) "I choose Peace" before you enter any dialogue or action.

It may feel silly at first. It may feel artificial or mechanical. Just remember this technique is only needed in the beginning of the process of becoming a Peace manager. It will very soon become automatic for you.

Reflect on your use of this technique:

Technique: Academy Award Winner

This is an easy technique to use early in the process of becoming a Peace manager. It is not a technique I advocate that you use often or as you become more skilled. The reason is that, although it may work for you in preventing a charge, it can still create chaos to which the other people around you, who may not be skilled Peace managers, will react. Our eventual goal is to be a Peace manager and also to promote peace all around us. As Peace becomes the way you are, the Academy Award winner will only be used on rare occasions, if at all.

As the title implies, this technique requires becoming a good actor or actress. This means you may use the words, tone of voice, or gestures that are an exaggeration of your true feelings, simply for the purpose of making a point. It is a conscious decision to communicate in this style, after having made the choice in the first tier, that of choosing to come from a place of Peace.

Let's go back to the example of getting the kids ready for bed. You may not be in a very creative mode and may not want to put forth the effort to try a more subtle approach to motivating the children. You can decide to maintain your Peace, but you can talk to your children in your traditional mother or father voice, point your finger boldly, and firmly tell them the consequences. To them, it will still sound like you mean business as much as you did the night before. You will sound and act the same, but you know the difference—no stress, just Peace.

Like I said, a more gentle approach might be more beneficial in the long run, but sometimes we simply don't have the time or energy to go the extra mile. Just make the gentle approach an eventual goal.

I am a very experienced Peace manager (eight years in the making), and I admit sometimes I still resort to this technique. It is a good one to have in your repertoire. I might need to make my son speed up his process for leaving the house when we are expected to be someplace at a specific time. I might start out with a gentle approach, but as all experienced parents know, we sometimes have to get more firm.

I use the old-fashioned phrases, quasi threats, raised voice, and sharp gestures. (Can you see why it is not ideal?) They work in motivating my son and maintaining my Peace. But I am sure he experiences a bit of guilt, frustration, and stress. This is not my goal. I feel much more successful when I say, "just so you know, I am not going to raise my voice, but I am serious about this. We need to leave the house in two minutes."

Whenever I do utilize the Academy Award winner, I usually get the same reaction out of my son, which leads me to the next topic. He usually says something like "I thought you were the Peace management Queen." I also have my standard reply, "I don't have a charge. How about you?" And yes, I get *that look*.

What does that phrase mean, and how can I tell if I really have a charge or not? I am very, very aware of what my charge feels like. I can identify it instantly. But I also have a double check technique, called a "charge check". Remember, a charge is the autonomic nervous system's response to a thought. Can I turn off the autonomic nervous system at my will? No!

How do I perform a charge check? This concept was first introduced in "Change the Thought", but now let's apply it as a little experiment. Sit quietly, not allowing *any* thought to enter your mind. Ask yourself to attempt to feel stress or anger. While in that state of having no thoughts, can you make yourself feel stress or anger? The correct answer is "no." Remember the emotion of stress is your body's reaction to a thought. Well, it is the same in reverse. If the chemicals are out there in response to your autonomic nervous systems command, you cannot bring these chemicals back to baseline immediately.

Therefore, if you are really stressed and are saying angry, loud words and you stop mid way, you will still feel the surge of chemicals. Your body and mouth might have stopped, but the chemicals still circulate and work for a while. It feels as though you are internally revved up or racing on the inside. That is the double check technique; the charge check.

Remember, you must be honest with yourself. I might sense that one of my students is stressed in response to an experience we are sharing (possibly preparing for a procedure we will be performing on a patient, or a need to talk to the nurse manager). If I ask them if they have a charge, they sometimes answer "no." Then I ask them to be honest. They give me that look, knowing I know something. I respond with something like "that blotchy red neck doesn't appear when you don't have a charge. It is a response to the chemicals circulating in your body." Yes, you are the only one who really knows, but even if you can't be honest with others, at least be honest with yourself.

As far as Peace management goes, you are even allowed to swear (but not in front of the children), as long as there is no charge.

Use this technique with discretion. The shared moment not only belongs to you, it belongs to the other person as well.

<u>Exercise (I)</u>:

Academy Award Winner

Goals for this section:

- Utilize the technique of the Academy Award Winner when appropriate
- Develop the ability to use the double check technique as a way to monitor if you have a charge when attempting to utilize this technique

---

<u>Activity A:</u>

Practice using the technique when you see it is an appropriate option.

<u>Activity B:</u>

Next time you choose Peace, then utilize the Academy Award Winner technique, stop before you were intending to end the discussion and determine if you feel Peace or a rush of chemicals making you feel revved up. This will allow you to evaluate if you were an Academy Award Winner or if you were having a true emotional response.

Technique: Judging Hurts ***You***

I find it odd that strangers judge my clothes. (They're in style, they're pretty, they're ugly.) More odd than that . . . people judge *me* by my clothes. Stop and think about that for a moment.

When I go in to the corner store, it is always the same me. However I get very different reactions if I go in with
my grass-stained yard clothes, or
a crisp, white nurse's uniform, or
a slinky, beaded gown.

I once heard a saying, supposedly from Buddha, that went something like this:

You are not punished *for* your anger, you are punished *by* your anger.

I would like to take this concept and apply it to judging or being judgmental. I have never talked with anyone who thinks of themselves as "judgmental." Yet we all are, without even realizing it. Some are more overtly judgmental than others. That may be why we don't think of ourselves as being judgmental, because we are nothing like Aunt Sally. But it is our nature to interpret things to which we are exposed. Personally, I don't know anyone who experiences an event and views it as just that, an event. They give some interpretation to it. And I don't know many people who can leave it at simply interpreting what they see or are exposed to, either. Most take it to the next level and categorize it as something good or bad, evil, odd, kind, etc. Based on our previous experiences or values, we give everything in our existence some qualitative label, attempting to categorize it into something desirable or undesirable.

This judging is an activity that robs our Peace, and no one is doing that to you, but you! There is no one else involved in this. It is easy to blame another person for robbing your Peace when we get into a confrontation or a power play with another. However, judging goes on inside you. It is your own mind's creation.

I have grown to appreciate the time I spend alone in my car. I live in the country, but I work in the city. Therefore, I have plenty of car time. This is where I learned to practice and incorporate many of these techniques. While I am driving, I might see an older man getting his mail. Rather that just observing him at face value, allowing my senses the intake (meaning simply staying at the level of awareness), I begin to think. First, I might label him as "old." In the reference library in my head, I categorize old age as undesirable. I then begin with the drifting thoughts. I might start thinking about my own aging and where that leads to, what changes I might experience as I age, and the limitations of movement I may have ahead of me. All this started because I labeled a man as old.

Can you see how we are punished *by* our judgment, not *for* our judgment. I punish my mind and spirit and eventually my body (being in the absence of Peace), as I focus on the fact that there are things that are desirable and things that are not.

There are three approaches you can choose to take. I am not going to advocate any one technique, as I alternately utilize all three. First, you can choose to work toward not allowing your mind to judge, remaining focused on the sensory intake. This is actually fun and allows you to really experience the Moment (or the "Now" as described by Eckhart Tolle). This is something I enjoy working on, but by no means can I do it on a regular basis and at a subconscious level. (Some of these techniques will be presented in exercise format, but for a more in-depth look at this, I recommend Tolle's book, *The Power of Now*.) I still must practice purposefully engaging in this first approach to limiting judgment. My hope is that someday I will do this automatically. If I stay in the Moment, just looking, listening, smelling, feeling, or tasting, there is no judgment, just experience. Once I label and critique, I am now in the place of judgment. This makes me realize I am in a place of "lack" or could potentially experience that place of lack. This sets off that downward spiral in my head, which robs my Peace.

For me, remaining nonjudgmental means driving down the road with the intent to *see* the new buds on the trees or the man walking down his drive, *hear* the wind outside or the sound of car horns, or *smell* the freshly cut grass or the smell of cow manure. Never giving any of it any meaning, just enjoying (yes, even the cow manure).

The second approach is to catch yourself in the moment of judging and realize this is detrimental to your Peace, and eventually, to your health. You then need to release the judgment, realizing that it is not possible from your vantage point to judge whether something is good or bad. You will have the opportunity to practice this awareness in the next exercise. It is arrogant of me to think I know what is good or bad in the big picture. When people make judgments based on limited information, that is arrogance. All judgments are based on limited information, because none of us are all-knowing.

Third, if you have difficulty giving up judgment altogether, attempt to look only at the positive side of the coin. This is fairly artificial, but can be used as a last resort. I admit that there are still times in my life when I must use this technique. Unexpectedly, I was exposed to a young man in my community who had a very disfigured face. Right away my mind carried me away with thoughts of pity, "what if it were me…" and fear of coming into unexpected contact with him and trying to hide my reaction again. This thought process truly robbed my Peace, possibly more than anything else in my life. Part of the issue was that running into this person caught me so off guard that my initial reaction was one of shock and horror. He was aware of my reaction. Our subsequent conversation was very awkward and unnatural. I kept thinking, I am a nurse, I shouldn't have handled this situation in this manner. In this instance, I even judged myself.

My husband and my best friend tried offering suggestions during the two weeks after this incident, when I was intensely robbed of my Peace. I was consumed with judgmental thoughts as I went to bed, first thing when I woke up in the morning, and throughout the day. I was well aware of the fact that I was not at Peace, but this situation really stumped me. The only thing that finally took me out of a place of judgment and Peace-lacking thoughts about the situation and the man's appearance was thinking "how could I, in the big picture know that this man's disfigurement is a bad thing." (This was using the technique to look at the positive.)

On the surface, the man's disfigurement was a very bad thing. But the more I looked at his situation, I thought back to our interaction and I began to see what an incredible person this young man was, probably in part because of what he had had to endure. I began to see that I was only looking at a very small piece of the picture. Disfigurement is not something that many of us would choose to experience if we had the choice. However, after noting his grace, maturity, and level of self confidence, I saw that it had obviously served him well.

On a smaller scale, when you think about the old man, try to think about the positive side. The charge we are trying to eliminate to promote our health is not from the positive emotions, it is from the negative ones. Instead of thinking about the fact that he has limited movement, think of the sufficient mobility he had to get to the mailbox. He may be very proud of his mobility. It may bring him extreme joy. Or it may make you focus on things like bringing yoga body exercises into your routine, drawing your focus to that, rather than on the lack of mobility.

Realize this third approach is not eliminating judging, but it is "going in the back door" solely for the purpose of eliminating a charge. Therefore, it is not the best technique, but it is one you can use in the process. It is better not to judge at all, but if this is not possible, you need to at least change your focus, to steer away from the snowball effect that the meaning behind the judgment has for you.

One student told me about a form of judgment of which I was not aware. Some people in the black community judge the quality of another black person by the amount of dark pigmentation they have in their skin. How it was conveyed to me was that some black people value other black people more if they don't have as much pigment in their skin. (The lighter shades of brown are more desirable).

This is a concept that, I must say, shocked me, especially when I learned how it played out in one young woman's life. Lonna stated that she was rejected by her light skinned, black grandmother because of the darkness of her skin. Lonna has a medium shade of brown skin. Lonna has two sisters, one very light skinned and one "just a shade lighter" than Lonna.

The grandmother has bonded and "bent over backwards" for the other two sisters, but essentially shuns Lonna. I have interacted on a deep level with many people in my life. I have to say that Lonna has a very kind and gentle spirit. She is one of the most loving and hard-working women I know. I can't help but think that the grandmother hurt herself by not allowing herself the opportunity to intimately know such an incredible, loving human being. Lonna's grandmother is not punished *for* her judgment, she is punished *by* her judgment.

At this point, I feel it is important to mention the difference between judging for the sake of judging (being judgmental) and judging as a step in the decision making or problem solving process. The Peace robbing judging I have explained above serves no real purpose for you. Yes, it adds to your brain's inventory of values and desires, but that clutter is not needed for your daily activities or for enriching your life.

However, when it comes to making a decision or solving a problem, you will in a sense be judging if something is right for you or not. I refer to this form of judging as "evaluating." The judging is not the focus of the decision making process. It happens in a very "behind the scenes" kind of way. You already know what is right for you at a deep level. This whole topic is presented in more detail in the section entitled *Listen to your Gut.*

This concept and set of techniques may be the hardest one for you. It was (and is) for me. I am continually trying to heighten my awareness of my judgments. I have asked people close to me not to use judgmental words, as I feel that when I am surrounded by prejudices or judgmental attitudes or words this sabotages my attempt to stay judgment-free. I also try to bring my conscious awareness to this matter at every opportunity. I am much better and much more Peaceful in this area, but I have a long way to go.

Exercise (J):

Eliminate the Tendency to Judge

Goals for this section:

- Increase your awareness of the frequency with which you are judging
- Employ techniques to transform moments from a state of judging to a state of experiencing
- Realize the difficulty and futility of determining if something is good or bad
- Determine the benefits to you of being without judgment, and examine the toll it places on you to be in a place of judgment

---

Activity A:

The next time you are in a car or going about your daily business (either in a store, at work, or any other place you choose), make a purposeful attempt to be aware of your thoughts and how frequently judgment comes into play.

Try to follow your train of thought once judgment has entered the picture.

When you were in that place of judgment, what did you feel in your body?

Activity B:

After you complete Activity A, again be aware of your judgments. But this time, make a conscious effort to stay in the experiencing mode.

Simply look, listen, feel, smell, and taste. Do not give these sensory experiences any label, any meaning, or think about them in terms of being good or bad.

Would you call it Peace when you were experiencing life and your surroundings this way?

What did you feel in your body?

Activity C: Flip Flop Game

Time to play a little game. This exercise serves the point well. All you need to do is carry the *Flip Flop Game* a few steps to get the picture, but try it on a few examples/story lines.

For the sake of the game, I will label things as good or bad, but realize this portion of the game is even counter-productive in the big picture.

The object here is to take a stand on something as good or bad, but then quickly think of the opposite effect that could come of the situation.

Here goes my example:

Oh no, I am late for work.
(bad thing)

→

Because I am late for work, I didn't have to deal with the project manager who would ask me if I will meet my deadline tomorrow.
(good thing)

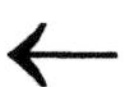

Because I didn't talk to the project manager, I didn't know that we made several changes we need to take into account before we finalize the proposal.
(bad thing)

→

Because I didn't know about the changes my manager wanted me to make, I continued on my plan. The client ended up liking my idea, and our team won the bid.
(good thing)

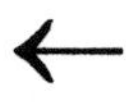

I upset my boss because I did not know about his new plan, and even though that lack of knowledge is what won the bid, he had me moved to another project team.
(bad thing)

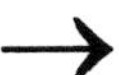

Because I got moved to a new project team, I had more visibility with the Department Chair and got a huge raise and promotion.
(good thing)

Try this exercise with your own real or created situation. Once you begin doing this, you become very clear that nothing is inherently bad or good. It is simply bad or good because of the meaning that we attach to it.

Again, a brief reminder that it would be very arrogant to think that in my very small world, from my very limited perspective in life, I judge something as good or bad.

Activity D:

Take a moment to write down your reflection on this exercise and on this way of thinking, if this is a new concept for you:

How does it feel *not to come from* a place of judgment?

How does that feel in your body?

Would you describe this as Peace?

Technique: Lose the "I'd Rather Be Right than at Peace" Attitude

This is possibly the second time in this program you will experience having your shackles shaken. And I know it doesn't feel good initially. I was not a fan of this part of the process either. But now, I actually welcome someone who challenges me to take experiencing Peace to the next level. So, this discomfort from shackle shaking only lasts momentarily for me. It is just the initial phase that doesn't feel good. Once the shackles are shaken, I then feel the motivation necessary to break free.

I have found that the process of *breaking past* thoughts and ideas that hold me back or hold me down, helps in my growth. In fact, having someone challenge me to assist with breaking free from my shackles became one of the mandatory components of relationships with men I was dating. I believe that most women, when seeking a mate, look for things like financial stability, sexual chemistry, or shared goals. Although I think those are important, I find it more important that my partner in life lovingly challenges me to always be a better me. Our tendency otherwise is to stay in our comfort zone, no matter how dysfunctional it is. For Peace to become the mainstay of our existence, we must be willing to break free from the things that hold us back. You can do this process on your own. However, you move through the process of attaining regular Peace faster when someone else helps bring it to the forefront of your mind.

Well, here goes. The first shackle shaking technique I presented was "Release the Drama Queen." Do you remember how uncomfortable it was to admit that *possibly* you were a part of some drama in your life? If you are like most, once you got that concept, you became acutely aware that most of the fights you get in have a bit of drama to them. You might also have begun to notice the drama in situations and relationships around you. And most importantly, you began to notice how engaging in drama actually robs your Peace.

We all engage in personality-specific traits that create shackles. You will have an opportunity to analyze your own tendency to shackle yourself in a later section. The reason this personality trait is separated out is that like the Drama Queen, I feel we all have a little bit of this in us.

You already know the title of this technique. (In case you forgot, look at the top of this section. Don't make me run my nails on the chalkboard again). And yes, this Peace robber pertains to you, too. I have yet to find a person who doesn't have the desire to be viewed as right. When I ask this question, about the need to be viewed as right, to groups, I never get anyone to say they never experience this need. For some reason, people are honest with this one.

The title of this technique is fairly self explanatory. There is no place for arrogance in Peace. So what this means is that there will be very few instances where proving that you are right is more important than the Peace that the two individuals lose during the discussion of who is right.

Now, I am not saying this applies to things like where to put a post when building a bridge or deciding about taking out an organ during surgery. I do want 100% accuracy with these decisions. And it would be appropriate to present your case in an effort to persuade. But in the upcoming book *Peace management in the Workplace* we actually discuss how to work through professional disagreements while maintaining your Peace and actually promoting the Peace of others.

Here, the attitude of "I'd rather be right than at Peace" is addressed in terms of personal growth. And I think you know the type I am talking about. I'm sure that at one time or another you have been in a conversation or argument that lasted much longer than it should have, because both people involved were certain they were right. Hurtful words may even have been exchanged, just because each was willing to go to any extreme to prove they were right. So rather than the individuals spending the time and energy on figuring out how to fix what was wrong, they wasted all their energy proving that they were right. Thinking back, were any real solutions found, and did both of you lose your Peace? Isn't memory of futile arguments enough to make you willing to reconsider your insistence on being right?

I think when we stop to realize that minimal benefits are derived from many debates, it is easy to see that choosing Peace is much more beneficial. You could choose to waste your time proving you are right. Each of you could probably recruit armies to support your side. For what gain?

A quote I heard years ago speaks to this whole concept in a different way:

"Blame is easier than guilt."

I agree, but neither is the way to go. It simply explains one reason that people may be so ardent in their need to be right.

Choosing Peace over the need to be right goes a step beyond "let's agree to disagree." When we choose Peace in potentially argumentative situations, we switch the focus and simply see that someone disagrees with us. It is an opportunity for us to grow and expand our thinking. We realize that there is another way to think about this issue. Choosing Peace doesn't mean I need to agree with the other person at all, and definitely not in this moment, but it enables me to know there are other ways of thinking about an issue than mine.

If you can get out of the mode of trying to persuade others to accept your point of view (how could I know what is right for them) and simply approach discussions as if they are mind-expanding forums, not only will you end up being an open thinker, but you will have Peace. You will no longer feel you have to prove you are right or defend your stance, and you will not waste energy on developing the strategy to prove you are right. I experience a prolonged exhale just thinking about this new type of communication mode.

In instances where you are communicating a difference of opinion, stay focused on why it is right for *you* and *why* you are making the decision. Do not change the focus to attempt to persuade the other person. This is what could lead to the battle of proving you are right. You may choose to acknowledge that the other person has valid input that would go into the decision if he/she were faced with the same situation. However, this acknowledgment is not necessary.

One other concept that I would like to present here, before you move on to the exercise, is the value of using stress management or anger management techniques to get you back to a baseline so that you are able to manage Peace. Hopefully, by this point in the program you are very clear that Peace management is not a new form of anger management or stress management. Hopefully, it will actually make stress management and anger management classes obsolete. But this does not mean they do not have their place. Especially while you are a new Peace manager, you will experience many episodes of stress or anger. My hope here is that you at least recognize the stress early in the experience. Once you recognize it, you know that stress or anger is there. This is not a time to manage your Peace. You can't! You are not in Peace. So you can't manage it. You have to be in a place of Peace to manage it. If you are not at Peace, you must resort to stress management or anger management. Remember, both of these strategies are too late for the sake of health and well being. The health-eroding chemicals are already out there doing their damage.

Therefore, when you realize you are experiencing stress or anger, you must use some strategy of stress management or anger management to get you back to Peace, because you value coming from a place of Peace. When you realize you are not in a place of Peace, step back and use some form of stress management or anger management. Some ideas might be relaxation techniques or distraction. Once you are back to Peace, tell yourself "I am not going back there again. I will continue this discussion from a place of Peace." Now you are managing Peace. Our eventual goal is to need only the skills of Peace management, because we will never go to stress or anger.

It is time to begin looking at your own need to be right. In a later technique where we analyze personality traits, you will understand how difficult it is to deal with perceptions. So for the sake of this exercise, simply admit that "having a need to be right" is one of your characteristics and have a willingness to release it for the benefit of experiencing Peace and promoting peace in a relationship.

Exercise (K):

I'd Rather Be at Peace

Goals for this section:

- Identify the fact that, at least occasionally, you have a strong need to be right at almost any cost
- List the areas that have created the strongest urge for you to be right
- Analyze the presence of a relationship between conversations when you feel a need to be right and the resulting loss of Peace
- Determine if it is worth releasing the need to be right for the benefit of experiencing Peace within yourself and in a relationship

---

Activity A:

Take a moment to determine if you have ever experienced a strong need to be right. How strongly do you feel about issues where you believe you are right? Are you willing to use multiple strategies and approaches to convince the other person that you are right?

Activity B:

List all the areas that you defend strongly, and where you may try to convince others that your stand is the correct stand or approach:

1. ____

2. ____

3. ____

4. ____

5. ____

Activity C:

Replay the possible dialogue of the conversations you might have had in relation to each item on your list in Exercise B. Try to relive the feelings you experienced.

Do you remember any feelings of anger or stress during these conversations?

Do you equate the feelings of stress, frustration, or anger to a loss of Peace?

Activity D:

Are you willing to try working through differences of opinion from a place of Peace? I am not talking about giving in for the sake of stopping an argument; that is passive or an act of avoidance. Rather I am talking about an active choice for Peace.

In addition to Peace, what other benefits may come about from choosing to discuss differences from a place of Peace?

Technique: Acknowledge the Suffering

Peace is our natural and intended state. Yet, by our choices and our reactions, we allow ourselves to be diverted to a place that lacks Peace. Anyone or anything that overtly or insidiously robs our Peace is toxic to Peace. The concept of toxicity will reappear later.

"Acknowledge the Suffering" is peripherally a part of the Peace management program. It is not directly a technique in Peace management, yet it is a concept that deserves our attention because suffering can interfere with becoming a true Peace manager. Suffering must be dealt with as part of the process, as this is something that robs Peace.

Acknowledging the suffering is part the process intended to identify and address things that *block* your ability to achieve Peace. It is unlike many of the other techniques, which are intended to maintain Peace or prevent you from going to a place that lacks Peace. It is intended more to serve the purpose of "acknowledging" in an effort to identify the presence of suffering. This will prepare you to attempt various techniques to allow Peace to resume its natural presence.

Suffering is the emotional burden we carry in relation to a physical experience or life event. It is what causes us the distress of the experience. It is what we emotionally attach to something. Suffering is a large component of what nurses encounter in their interactions with patients. Most nurses understand suffering at their core, from repeated contacts and struggles. Yet, when I tried to research suffering in my nursing books, there was surprisingly little in print. This indicates it is a concept that deserves more exploration and attention.

Suffering is best illustrated with an example. This is the exact example I use when teaching my nursing students. I say to them,

> If you injured your hand and ended up missing the ends of a couple of fingers, and I asked you to rate your pain on a scale of 1 - 10 (10 being the most pain), you might answer "6." Now if you were a professional piano player and I asked you the same question, you might say a "12." The physical sensation may be no different, but the suffering associated with the physical experience magnifies the physical pain.

My students and I experienced a real life situation that illustrates the impact of suffering. We cared for a very attractive woman who was in a traumatic accident and required an amputation of her left leg, just below the knee. This happened after several painful and futile operations attempting to save the limb. The staff nurses were not able to get her pain under control, no matter how much medication they gave to her. They even consulted Pain Management services to attempt to bring relief. We decided to talk to her about her pain. In our conversation, we found out that she was a professional ballroom dancer who competed regularly. Need I say more?

As a society we do acknowledge that there is a difference between pain and suffering. In fact, a phrase we use says just that: pain *and* suffering. The "and" suggests they are two separate concepts. Or you might hear the term "suffers from allergies." This phrase does not refer to the actual symptoms or pain (running nose, burning, or itching eyes). It refers to the impact it has on your life.

I work with students and new nurses regularly. They ache for their patients and are quick to give pain medications. Although I also tend to liberally medicate my patients for pain, I simultaneously attempt to inquire about the meaning of the pain for them. This helps me utilize the appropriate measures to bring about relief. I also utilize Peace management and request counsel from other healthcare professionals to assist in total care for my patients.

So far, I have focused on the suffering that is attached to physical pain or ailment. Yet suffering can be the emotional burden that is attached to other types of losses, changes, or undesirable situations. For example, people who experience events such as divorce, loss of a child, or getting fired also experience some form of suffering.

An easy example to begin understanding this is the suffering that is experienced in relation to a miscarriage. The parents are essentially grieving over the loss of someone whom they did not even know in this physical world. Yet there is intense suffering at times. What is this all about? It is about experiencing the loss of what that person or situation meant to the prospective parents or grieving the loss of what might have been. It is the meaning they attached to the loss.

With a miscarriage, a couple may be suffering as they experience the loss. They may have lost that potential feeling of a family and all the things they might have been planning to do with that child, or the dreams they had for that child. If there are no other children, this miscarriage means they are still "childless," which can bring up a whole new set of issues that cause suffering.

When your baseline of experience is not a deep sense of Peace, it is important to look at the potential that you may be experiencing some suffering. I could not even begin to include a laundry list of the things that may be causing your suffering. You need to go within yourself and see if you are carrying an emotional burden related to some situation or event. This may be a hard exercise, because you may be acknowledging things you would rather keep swept under the carpet. Yet it will be very important because suffering may be one of the biggest things robbing your Peace.

After taking my son to school, I came home to find a note from my husband. It read:

Your mom called
she had heart palpitations all night
long. Call her. Wants to know if she
should go to the Doctor.

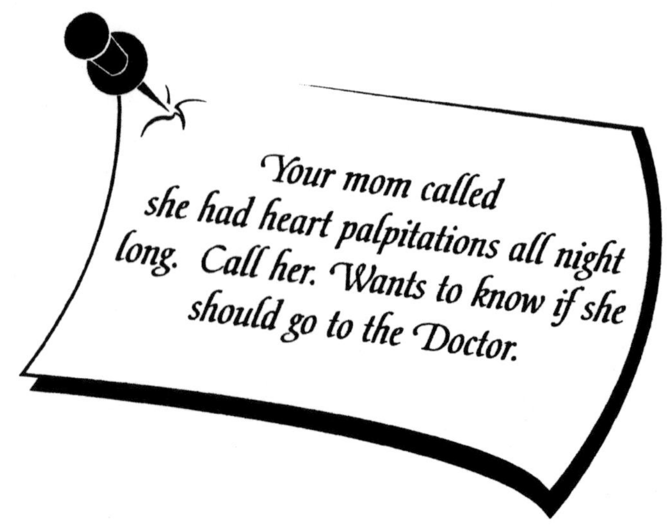

When I called my mother, she started right in with answers to questions I had not even asked yet. I guess that when you are the mother of the person writing Peace management, you know what your daughter first considers with any health disorder. She started out by saying, "your father and I had a very relaxing evening last night, and nothing out of the ordinary happened." I realized she didn't want me to discuss the effects of stress, so I started asking my other typical questions: "Did you have coffee last evening? Do you feel any other kind of illness or pain? Did you have more activity than normal?" The answers were all "no." Yet I still felt there was something "fixable" going on. I decided to pursue my instinct.

A light bulb went on for me. I said "you and dad had a relaxing evening, doing relaxing things? What did you do?" My mom said, "We went for a long dinner, took a walk, then just came home and sat outside." I realized that those activities probably provided her with an abundance of quiet time. I knew what my mom had been struggling with lately.

Right on the heels of the death of her own mother, she had suddenly lost a young cousin, with whom she felt very connected. Also, someone very dear to her was dying of a devastating illness, and the husband of a close friend was losing a long battle with cancer. In fact, two days before, my mother had called to tell me the doctor had informed the couple that the cancer had "exploded" inside the man's body. I wish that pictorial choice of words had not been used, but that was the doctor's explanation, and now we were all dealing with the fall out of that image.

Knowing all of this, I asked my mom "What was on your mind during these relaxed moments?" Well, you guessed it. She had spent most of the time thinking about all of these losses and potential losses in her life. She knew in her heart what had brought on the palpitations. I think she felt badly that she let her grief get the best of her, because she was well aware of Peace management. She said to me, "I need to talk to you because I need to have you help me get my Peace." She knew that she needed to get a handle on her sense of loss.

Together, we approached getting in touch with the problem from a point of suffering. We were able to label some of the meaning that the losses represented to her:

her own mortality
she won't have Maria to talk to or share life experiences with
she lost her maternal nurturer
she cannot fill the hole that her dad will certainly experience
the potential for many other losses.

I asked my mom to spend the rest of the day getting in touch with the meaning of these loses that she had identified and the suffering she was experiencing, so that we could move forward. One technique I hope to move her into shortly is called "Go There." This will allow her to experience the feelings that she is pushing away, while she will be in a very controlled place. This technique has the ability to take away the pain that anticipation carries. My mother's mind is swirling with thoughts about the past and the future. Both types of thoughts are having an impact on her present. She is carrying an emotional burden, or suffering now.

A major point that I would like to make here is that it is not your body being in a relaxed state (although you will see that I advocate this) nor a relaxing environment (and I also advocate this) that is the main focus of Peace management. I will present some of these peace promoters later. The main focus of Peace management is *controlling your mind*. As I told my mother, she could have been sitting on a quiet beach by herself, and her Peace could have been robbed. The "relaxing evening" only helped mask what had caused her palpitations.

In the presence of suffering, there is no Peace. They are mutually exclusive. They cannot co-habitate a moment in time. It is one or the other. We need to "acknowledge" suffering, because the management of suffering is, in a sense beyond the reaches of Peace management. That is not to say that people suffering cannot use Peace management. On the contrary, you can choose Peace in any moment. Yet suffering is an underlying experience that can rob you of your Peace. You must realize that if you are having trouble experiencing Peace, it may be due to some suffering you are experiencing. You need to specifically identify the suffering and analyze what it means to you.

Once you look at the meaning, you might then want to explore ways to minimize the suffering, until it is absent from your existence. It is easier to just choose Peace in the moment, but I realize each of you has your own story, full of various levels of suffering which have lead you to become the current you. Therefore, you can choose Peace in every new moment, or you can choose to at least acknowledge that you are suffering. If you choose to simply start by acknowledging the suffering, as a way to move gradually toward experiencing more Peace, this is acceptable The choice is yours.

In trying to acknowledge the suffering, you must realize the suffering is the meaning the event or circumstance takes on for *you*. You must label it appropriately before you can begin working through it. You can not take on suffering for someone else. As you might have noticed, when we started labeling the areas of suffering that my mom was experiencing, they were worded as the meaning they had for *her*.

This possible confusion came to light for me when working with a student. Fran said that she suffers for her children because their dad (her ex-husband) does not show that he cares for the children. She said their father will tell the children he is going to spend some time with them or buy them a gift for their birthdays, but he never does. The children get very sad. Fran said she suffers for them. I felt I needed to have her experience labeled correctly so she could begin working on it and also assist her children in their work.

Fran cannot suffer *for* her children. Fran can try to understand what they are going through and have sadness about the situation. Fran can suffer because of the meaning she attaches to this situation. The children can suffer as a result of the meaning they attach to the situation. Let's break these sentences down to explore the complexity of this concept:

Fran can try to understand what the children are going through and have sadness about the situation.

Fran can listen to her children's comments or understand them through relating them to her children's prior history and coping. She can feel sadness as she understands human vulnerability and how people experience loss or disappointment.

Fran can suffer because of the meaning she attaches to this situation.

Fran can attach some meaning to the experience, which can create her own sense of suffering. When I explored this with Fran, she was able to identify the meaning this situation had for her. She said it was the fact that she didn't have the ability to provide everything her children needed to be happy. She felt suffering for not having the ability to make the situation better. She also felt some guilt for having had a hand in the decision to divorce, which caused the situation of the children's father not being in their life on a regular basis. (And as a side note: this is not a time to judge the validity of your feelings. Fran could have rationalized that she really did not have a hand in the decision of the divorce, that it was beyond her control. But this would only make it more difficult to label the meaning behind the feeling she is calling suffering.) Fran successfully labeled what caused her the emotional burden in relation to this situation.

The children can suffer as a result of the meaning they attach to the situation.

Fran explored this with her children. Her children were able to label the emotional burden, or the meaning of the experience, as "not being good enough or not behaving well enough so that their father would want to be with them or buy them a birthday gift." They felt like they were not important to someone whom they felt should make them important. That caused them to suffer.

This process started this family on their way to understanding their feelings. Fran expressed that they all felt "lighter" as they were able to understand "what dragged them down." They are now moving ahead as a family and each of them are individually working toward becoming Peace managers.

If this concept of "acknowledging the suffering" touched you deeply, you may want to move forward to "take charge of sadness." Otherwise, simply being aware of this concept may assist you in removing this block, should it arise for you.

<u>Exercise (L)</u>:

Acknowledge the Suffering

Goals for this section:

- Identify any areas that could be labeled as suffering (the emotional burden you are carrying related to an event or situation).
- Analyze the meaning behind the circumstance that creates the feeling of suffering.
- Begin any attempts to make a commitment to yourself to eventually eliminate suffering

---

<u>Activity:</u>

Whenever you are in a moment that feels like the absence of Peace, examine if there are any components of suffering that are robbing the potential for Peace.

What are those areas:

(you may want to use your deck of cards to begin creating this list)

What is the associated *meaning* behind these circumstances that creates the feeling of suffering:

If you truly value Peace, make a commitment to allow yourself to explore the possibility that you are suffering. Identify if suffering is robbing your Peace.

Determine if you will allow the suffering to rob your Peace.

Technique: Cultivate Compassion

We all experience varying degrees of impatience and intolerance of others. This feeling inside of us robs our Peace. I use to be just as guilty as the next person of this tendency. Think back to your charge cards. Were any of your cards the label of a person? Mother, boss, sister-in-law? These "charges" most likely stem from your disapproval of the disparity between your values, choices, or actions and theirs.

A very effective technique for dealing with your loss of Peace in relation to a person is "cultivating compassion." I use the term cultivating, because, my guess is that you will not create an immediate 180° change in the relationship, although that is not entirely impossible. I have one student who comes to mind. She told me of the rapid and drastic change she had in relating to her mother-in-law, once she decided to approach her with compassion. And this is a woman who "drove her crazy daily," as she was the baby-sitter for her children while she attended school.

More often that not, my guess is that a change will happen gradually. This is how it has proceeded in my life and in the lives of most people I counsel. The word "cultivate" connotes a feeling of nurturing, laying the ground work, and caring about the improvement of the relationship. This will not only benefit the other person and the quality of the relationship, but it will also benefit you. You have an opportunity to experience Peace in formerly stressful interactions and relationships.

Most of the feedback I receive from my students reveals that the biggest causes of stress and anger in their lives are interactions with certain individuals. From my own life experience, I agree with my students. That is why cultivating compassion takes on such importance. I utilize this strategy often.

What is compassion? No dictionary can adequately describe this very complex concept. The best way to approach understanding compassion, in order to employ it as a technique, will be to look at it from various angles and examples.

One aspect of compassion is unconditional acceptance. We often hear about unconditional love. Well, this is a spin-off. The person in front of us, who may be driving us crazy, is a product of all their life experiences and life lessons. They simply are who they are. All people evolve into the "continually current me." Your "current you" is meeting the "current them." Two very complex beings, each with your own sets of values, beliefs, and morals. This makes for very complex interactions.

We can actually make this complexity very easy: I accept people for whom they are. Saying this, I must also include the warning that it is also wise to maintain boundaries. If I feel they invade these lines, I can gently and kindly make it known. I do not need to allow myself to feel that I am compromising my beliefs and needs, but I accept whom they are as an individual. I do not judge how or why they choose specific words or actions to communicate.

Remember, many people suffer for different reasons. People who try your patience may be acting in a way that is self-preserving, attempting to avoid any feeling of suffering. If we understand that, we can have acceptance and compassion for how they react. Compassion requires depersonalizing the interaction. This may seem to run counter to what your beliefs are about compassion. This involves not taking their reaction personally. There is no need to personalize how another individual responds to situations. It is simply their choice to react as they do. Compassion involves an understanding that others have different experiences and interpretations. You accept *them* without judgment, whether you accept the idea or not.

A potential conflict may arise if the other person attempts to exert their control to influence your thoughts or actions. You do not have to accept their suggestion if it does not fit your belief system, but Peace is possible when you accept them as a person, with feelings and attitudes that belong to them. The goal is to come from a place of compassion, rather than defensiveness. Realize that most people are doing the best job that they can with their current skills and history.

A technique that helps cultivate compassion is taking the focus off of yourself and placing attention on the other individual. You can have compassion for yourself, but the focus of this section is attaining Peace in relation to relationships with other individuals. A great example of this came to me from a friend. Steven is a very successful but very busy business owner who keeps very long hours. He called me to ask advice on a health concern of his mom's, but started out by asking "Are you practicing Peace?" "Always," was my answer. Steven had been introduced to the concept and seemed to have just taken off with it. I asked him how his Peace management was going. He decided to share a story with me. It was just what I needed to illustrate compassion.

Steven is in a second marriage. He has three teenagers from his first marriage and a two year old from his current marriage. Steven is about 50 years old. He said he had worked a 12 hour day and was just beat. Worse yet, he had to pick up his two year old son, Travis, from day care. Travis had also been away from home for 12 hours. When they finally got home, Steven said Travis was just not comfortable in his own skin. He cried to be picked up, he cried to be put down. He took his socks off, and he cried because he couldn't put them back on by himself. He tried to eat, but then he would throw away the food. Travis was miserable. So was Steven.

Steven realized he had been focusing on *himself* and how Travis was making *his* situation worse. In that moment, Steven realized he was not at Peace and that he and Travis were probably feeding off each other's stress, which was making the situation worse. Steven realized that he had had trouble with the long, tiring day, and he was an adult. Travis was two years old, probably feeling the same thing, but not capable of understanding why he was feeling so miserable. Steven felt immediate compassion for Travis. Steven went into the other room for 30 seconds to get to a place of Peace. He "felt totally different." He came back, picked up Travis, and went to a chair. It was clear to Steven that Travis now sensed his Peace. Steven said that Travis cuddled in his arms and was asleep in 10 minutes.

Compassion is, in a sense, a place of "allowing." It allows others to be who they are. It is the way that serves them well at this time, as dysfunctional as it may seem. Their evolvement as a person is simply where it is, like it or not. It actually feels good to "allow." It takes you out of feeling that you have to be judge and jury. You get to sit in the courtroom, just being a spectator.

Compassion allows you to realize that the other person is human. With being human comes faults, sorrows, ineffective ways of communicating, and a multitude of other deficiencies. As we know, no one is perfect. And ya know what? They don't have to be! Everyone is working on their own struggles, traveling their own path, and learning their own life lessons in this strange Earth classroom.

What you will soon learn is that cultivating compassion in your life is a process. At first, it is helpful to put yourself in someone else's shoes. But soon you will realize that compassion really has nothing to do with the words we call sympathy or empathy. That is the "old fashioned" version of the concept of compassion. The old strategies actually did not promote what is intended by compassion. Those strategies actually create a greater gap between individuals, not allowing the experience of union. Sympathy also puts me in a one-up position of "feeling sorry" for them. There is no room for arrogance of any type when coming from true compassion. Also, there also is no benefit in *feeling* their pain, that is common with sympathy.

With empathy, you try to put yourself in the other person's shoes in an effort to understand their emotions better by projecting your personality on to their situation. This concept has many erroneous lines of logic. In addition to the illogical nature of this technique, there is no need to deeply understand their emotions to have compassion for them. Trying to empathize moves the focus to attempting to understand the reason the other individual feels pain, which is not necessary for compassion.

You will experience a knowing or understanding, of sorts. I acknowledge what people tell me their struggles are, as their reality, and I support them as they move through them. Or, I don't know what their struggles are, but I do know they are human and a product of their life experiences. Either way, I accept people as they are and decide to have a relationship with the "current them."

I also could not guess where others are in their growth, even if they put it into words. They may be using a form of coping that does not allow them to describe their issues accurately, or they simply may not be capable of adequately or fully describing their issues. It is clear that it would be futile to attempt to understand them fully. Admit it: do you even fully understand yourself, let alone another?

I work with students on a vascular surgery division. Many of these patients are very ill and require amputations because of the progression of their vascular disease. I have experienced such a wide array of responses to the need for an amputation that I gave up trying to figure out what patients may be going through. Some patients have already been through so much pain, suffering, and draining of finances that they actually welcome an amputation as a way to "get back to their life."

In the past, I would attempt to help my students anticipate what the patient's emotional state might be and what issues they might be facing. Now, I don't say a word. I let my students figure out each patient on their own, then I help them employ the appropriate strategies.

When you do allow the other person to make their choices and live their life, you are moving to a higher point in your relationship. This means not offering your interpretation of their situation or telling them what you would do if you were them. This allows the real you to meet the real them. You now have a chance for a genuine relationship, when each person is allowed to be their genuine self.

Many people have either written or unwritten goals that they use to guide them through their life and decisions. This provides a conscious direction to life. I do use visual (picture) cues for material goals. However, my written goals are different from most people's. My written goals focus on *how* I want to be and *what* I want to contribute to life. In writing these out, I am very conscious of the need to allow others to be themselves.

In fact, one of my goals related to raising my son is written like this: I will not interfere with his life lessons, but I will be there to support him in any and every way he needs me. That support can be in the form of guidance, suggestions, or advice, but I will not interfere in the way he has to learn about himself, life, and other people. That is *his* work while he is here, not *mine*. There is also some benefit for me in this. I have the opportunity to intimately watch the very creative experience of another human being unfold and grow, rather than just seeing a repeat performance of my life.

Everyone has the same basic human needs. Other than the physiological needs (food, water, and air), we all have needs for safety, love, belonging, acceptance, and respect. When any one of those needs feel threatened, people often resort to very primitive and dysfunctional measures. For example, if someone feels they are not being respected, they usually don't simply ask for respect. They act out in a way that, in a sense, demands it in a very disguised manner. The person on the receiving end is often confused and responds to circumstances and actions they don't understand.

A topic that often comes up in study groups for "A Course in Miracles" is the concept that there is only love or a cry for love. If this is something you believe, it would be easy to understand why people sometimes act in confusing or exaggerated ways. If they truly are crying out for love, a very basic need, the manifestation may look very strange.

The final concept I would like to present in relation to cultivating compassion is reverence. Reverence is what should be felt in any union of two people who interact. This is a difficult concept for me to cover here, because I feel limited in my ability to explain it. Yet it is very important, so I will attempt it. I know from my own experience that my interactions and relationships with people would feel very empty if I did not come from a place of reverence.

I receive a new group of nursing students every five weeks. That format could promote very superficial or minimally meaningful relationships. However, I do not feel that those students are placed in my metaphorical lap for me to interact on a superficial level. The only way for me to approach meaning and to come from a place of compassion for who they are and what they bring to our interactions is through the framework of reverence. I wouldn't have it any other way.

Reverence is a concept I regard with such high esteem, a sacredness-of sorts. Therefore, I take much care in attempting to communicate this. To make this more difficult, it is based on my interpretation of quantum physics. This in and of itself is a very difficult topic!

In having this material reviewed by a chemistry professor, he said that getting deeply into quantum physics takes people away from the sacredness of the reverence. He felt that I could get deeply into electromagnetic fields or the molecular changes that occur when we relate to someone. Or I could present what changes occur at a cellular level when we experience things. I do not want to make this section into a science treatise. This is not my intention, yet I am at a true loss of how to convey the material to you without touching on quantum physics. So for sake of presentation, I will present this to you, then try to build it back up into the sacredness of the concept, allowing you to explore its meaning on your own.

Even quantum physicists often have trouble explaining their field because they don't use a language that most people could relate to and there aren't many prior theories known to the general public on which they could begin their explanations. The "old rules" don't apply here. So, from a place of humility, here goes . . .

Quantum physics is the study and explanation of the very, very, very small particles of our world. Let's back up. At one time, humans acknowledged they had bodies, because they could see them. But that's all that they could say really existed. Then someone had the idea one day to cut open the body. They saw it was made up of smaller, very different things. We now call those things "organs." Then someone developed microscopes and instruments to look at organs more closely. They could then see smaller, living things that we now call cells.

Later, scientists and researchers developed electron microscopes. They were then able to identify things smaller than the cells. And the cells are so small that they could not be seen with the naked eye. Scientists called these very tiny particles atoms. Then they began to label the parts of the atom. In the center of the atom is something called a nucleus. In the nucleus are protons and neutrons. Orbiting around the nucleus are tiny things called electrons.

The study of quantum physics is the study of even smaller things, (and I don't know if we can call them "things" when they get to this point). Scientists have some names for these current tiniest parts, but they really are beyond me. I have used Webster's dictionary to simply define some of these terms if you are interested, but it really isn't important that you have a real grasp of them. Remember: "knowing is the booby prize." This means that knowing about something like this is not the real prize. Knowing through experience is what matters. What is important will be taking these concepts from physics and applying them to reverence, after I present one more concept.

The terms below, coupled with the principals of how they interact and what they really are, is work left for the physicists.

gluon - a quantum of energy or massless particle postulated to carry the force that binds quarks together within subatomic particles

quark - any of six types of flavors of hypothetical particles, plus their antiparticles, postulated as the building blocks of hadrons, in order to theoretically explain the properties of hadrons

hadrons - any of a class of subnuclear particles, including the baryons and mesons, that interact strongly and are thought to be made up of quarks

Quantum physicists also use terms like "color force," "exchange particles," "inverse square," and "green/anti-blue." Can you see why I am not going there? The only reason for my inclusion of this information in the first place is to help you wipe out any preconceived ideas you may have—that you know how things work. No one knows exactly what we are made of or what is at the very tiniest or core of us.

Anyway, let's begin the process of application. Some quantum physicists and metaphysicists explain that everything, at it's smallest level, comes down to light, energy, potential, or intelligence of some sort. So, for the sake of discussion, let's say that everything at its smallest source is light. I get the chills when I think of the biblical line where God said "let there be light." Wow!

What this means is that you are, in a sense, a bunch of condensed, compacted light that is held together by skin. And the skin itself is just a bunch of condensed light. So what is to say that your light ends right at the outside edge of your skin? We share atoms and subatomic particles with the air and everything else. Try a little experiment. Rub your hands together hard and fast, several times. Then hold your hands a couple of inches apart, palms facing in. What do you feel? This gives you a idea of the energy around us. Hold on, I am getting to "reverence."

There is a Hindu greeting that easily relates sacredness to my interpretation of quantum physics. When Hindus acknowledge each other, they say "Nemaste." Loosely translated, this means the light that is in you, which is the same light that is in me, is acknowledged and honored. This gives a whole new meaning to the concept that we are all one. You hear many speak of this, or say we are all brothers, or we are all linked, or what hurts you hurts me. In light of the concepts behind quantum physics, coupled with the feeling of Nemaste, our connection is understood and appreciated at a new level.

Reverence, to me, is the sacredness of the gift of sharing a moment with another human being. Therefore it makes compassion, or coming from a place of compassion, a very worthwhile effort. Applying the above information is a strategy for feeling reverence. I again apologize for my feeble attempt to explain this. Please spend time with these rough ideas and make them your own, through experience. The minister at my wedding defined love as "the experience of union." This speaks loudly to the concepts of compassion and reverence.

Imagine what it would be like to be on the receiving end of compassion. Pretty good! It would be unconditional acceptance in all life circumstances. You would never feel like you had to prove anything or live up to anyone else's expectations. You could always be yourself and be loved for it. Okay, wake me up!

Exercise (M):

Cultivate Compassion

Goals for this section:

- Practice coming from a place of compassion when interacting with people whom you normally allow to rob your Peace
- Note that coming from a place of compassion toward others allows you to experience Peace

---

Activity A:

Go to your deck of charge cards and pull out all the cards that represent a specific person.

Turn the cards over, and one-by-one begin practicing viewing the people represented in them from a place of compassion.

Activity B:

Next time you get angry at someone unexpectedly, attempt to quickly tell yourself that they are human, with all their faults and shortcomings. They deserve your compassion, simply because they are human beings.

Identify if the mood and feeling of the interaction changes as you choose to come from a place of compassion.

Activity C:

After you have done your work with the charge cards and feel capable of interacting with someone whom you formerly allowed to rob your Peace, choose to interact with them as an experiment.

What did you find during that interaction? Did you feel Peace? Did the other person react any differently to you?

Technique: Remove Toxicity

It may seem odd to talk about removing toxicity from your life, including people and relationships, immediately following the discussion on "coming from a place of compassion." However, this order represents my view of the appropriate process. Your first attempt to experience Peace when dealing with people should be an attempt at cultivating compassion. However, when that fails after an honest attempt, another approach must be taken. You cannot have toxicity in your life when you are attempting to change your essence to one who experiences Peace consistently.

I know removing toxicity sounds harsh, yet the reactions I get from students when we work through this concept in class is that it is not as harsh as the name sounds. In fact, one student said, "you know how Einstein had those 'Ah ha moments?' Well our group had a 'Duh' moment when we read it together." They said they couldn't believe they never came up with this concept on their own. The reason I am concerned that it may sound harsh is that you may reject it before you give it your complete attention. Trust me that it is a concept worth your attention.

I am not suggesting divorcing your spouse or throwing the kids out into the street. It is a different situation when you live with the people you consider toxic to your Peace. If this is the case, these relationships go to the top of your priority list for working on Peace management.

I risk sounding harsh purely for the benefit it brings. I feel strongly about this. Removing toxicity refers to much more than just people. Many things can be toxic to your potential for Peace: environments, conversations, people, jobs, addictions, and so on. Again, I am not saying quit your job tomorrow, although a job change may be a necessary thing, as long as it doesn't threaten your financial security. Financial insecurity could also be detrimental to your

Peace. It is time to begin identifying those things that are toxic to your Peace.

The first time I was introduced to this idea was in a "letter from the editor" in a woman's magazine. I cannot remember the name of the magazine. But the gist of the letter was that sometimes we need to distance ourselves from toxicity. This editor had breast cancer. She said that after she recovered from the surgeries, completed her chemotherapy, regained a head of hair, and returned to her roles as mother, wife, and editor, she made some very dramatic changes in her life, the most important change being the removal of toxicity. I wish this woman knew how much she has made an impact on me, and possibly on people who read this book. Her message was well received and valued.

This letter from the editor started a whole new way of thinking for me. I was easily able to identify things and people who were toxic to me. After the birth of Peace management, I carried the idea of toxicity further to include an awareness of things that were toxic to my Peace.

I do not see removing toxicity as "running away from" especially when it comes to people. My intention was to distance myself temporarily, until I was a more skilled practitioner of Peace management. I never intended to remove them and the toxicity they caused for me permanently. In fact, the real test of how effective of a Peace manager I am is the successful reintroduction into my life of the people from whom I distanced myself early in my evolution as a Peace manager.

This process of reintroduction has already started to occur for me. It is happening on various levels, according to the level of toxicity I feel these people brought to me. There are some individuals I totally removed from my interactions, and we are now starting to have brief Peace-full encounters.

I have totally received back into my life other individuals I had placed at a physical or emotional distance. Another group of individuals might not even realize that I have seen them as toxic and was not capable of interacting with them. They may not even have noticed the relative absence of interactions between us. They may have just perceived it as the normal fading of relationships that often takes place on its own. Some of these people are back in my life; some are not. I do not have strong feelings about the need for these interactions, therefore, I just let nature run its course in these relationships.

There can not be any *resistance* on your part to allowing people whom you considered toxic back in to your life, which also could take on the flavor of avoiding them or shunning them. Any grain of resistance will still be experienced as a lack in Peace. And although you may not see it at this point, we really are trying to move toward total Peace all the time. If achieving total Peace is not possible, I don't want to know it. Because that is the goal I am striving to attain. I am always looking to take Peace to the next level in my life.

So, in choosing not to have someone back in your life, you must think of it as a passive choice, of sorts: not "I will not let them back in my life," or "I don't want them back in my life," but rather, "there is no real need for me to seek them out to have them rejoin my life at this time." But even if you do not see a real need to have a certain person back in your life, you still need to be prepared for that chance encounter. Make a clear decision that you will choose Peace.

As far as non-human threats of toxicity to Peace, I am also at various stages of reintroduction into my life. However, as far as toxic environments go, I don't think I will ever choose to reintroduce them. An example of this is a smoke filled bar. The toxicity to my Peace does not refer to the direct danger of the smoke on my physical health. That is only an unwanted side effect. It is the *thoughts* of the effects of the smoke on myself, my son, and my husband that robbed me of my Peace when I was in that type of environment. These thoughts do not allow Peace in that moment, therefore I see them as toxic. I really think I could go into a smoke filled bar now and control my thoughts to maintain Peace, but I simply choose not to go there.

There are a few other toxicities that I would like to give special mention to:

- A conversation may feel toxic to you. Once you become aware of it, realize that it is an opportunity to practice Peace. If you are not able to practice Peace, simply excuse yourself. Step away from the conversation and return to Peace. This removal of toxicity is only a temporary measure during the learning phase of Peace management. You will eventually be able to stay in the conversations without receiving a charge.

- Become aware that the workplace can be a breeding ground for toxicity. Many dynamics come into play that provoke stress or anger. If fact, my eventual intention is to partner with a social scientist and a business expert to finish writing the book "Peace Management in the Workplace"©. The foundation is there; it simply needs expert input from these fields. There is a definite need, as the work environment is a major source of stress and anger for many people. Begin your own analysis of toxicity in your work situation.

- Another area that could be considered toxic is the legal system. With the national divorce rate approaching 50%, many of us will find ourselves in this system. In fact, personal experience and the experience of many friends and students has shown me that the "legal" system or "justice" system are erroneous positive names for our court system. In fact, simply using those names creates certain expectations.

  When you enter this system feeling that legal outcomes or justice will be done, or that going this route will be the avenue to bring you resolution or some form of Peace, you may be in for a big let-down. If the expectation was not there when you entered the system, a great deal of anguish and disappointment can be avoided.

Many people devote hours of work and preparation, then enter the legal system confident that their cause will prevail, only to be disappointed and distressed if the results are not commensurate with their efforts and expectations. Remember, lawyers and courts do not have the same goal in mind that you do. They do not care about your "happily ever after." Lawyers get paid by the hour, regardless of outcome, and courts want you off their docket. Their goals are not the same as your goals.

My recommendation is to avoid the court system and lawyers at all cost. You are intentionally entering into an adversarial relationship. As a new practitioner of Peace management, you will be setting yourself up for difficult times and frustration with this one. (As a side note: if you are a practicing attorney, you truly need Peace management. This is your life day in, and day out, every day, all day. You need to be able to perform your job from a place of Peace so that the stress does not affect your health.)

I am acutely aware that because so many marriages fail many of you may enter into the court system to some extent. My recommendation is "the less, the better," even for experienced practitioners of Peace. I don't know *anyone* who said the court process was enjoyable or peaceful. On top of that, it is very costly, which may set you up for other situations requiring you to "practice Peace." The choice is yours, but I would caution you to weigh all the options before working with lawyers and the court system. Something very drastic would need to occur before I would subject myself to that again.

I do not intend to alienate lawyers, judges, or people that work in a court house. In fact, some of my dear friends, as well as my father, whom I love dearly and respect immensely is a lawyer. But my intention here is to promote Peace and emotional healing, which will eventually impact physical health. I cannot think of a system that is more adversarial, toxic, or detrimental to emotional health than the court system. I feel an obligation, of sorts, to devote some attention to this since I experienced the negative impact on my own Peace.

- Reducing or eliminating your exposure to the news is a way of eliminating toxicity. I speak from experience, saying that once I totally removed the exposure to the news from my day, I was overall more Peace-full. I listen to people all over, on break at work or even in the grocery store, discussing news stories from a place of fear. Their focus becomes so fear-based.

  Several years ago, I began reducing the amount of news that I watch, and I am proud to say I have been news-free since 1997. I joke with my father, yet he responds willingly. I ask him to tell me when the stamps go up in price and when the clocks change (when the dates arrive to accommodate Daylight Savings Time). I tell him that these are the only bits of information I need to be able to function in life. Somehow, through conversations with other people, I do find out other tidbits of information. Yet I must admit, none of these tidbits have really affected my day-to-day living, even the information that we are in for a blizzard. I have 4 wheel drive and I always leave very early for work. If you really do need other "important" information, there are multiple ways to access it without subjecting yourself to radio and television news broadcasts.

  Last summer our house was struck by lightening on July 7th. We lost our TVs, VCRs, portable phones, and the well pump for our water. The only one we replaced with speed was the well pump. It wasn't until after Christmas, when my son was feeling like he wanted to watch some TV on wintery Saturday mornings, that I paid a visit to the electronics super store. We never missed having a working TV. My son is very athletic-oriented, and spends most of his free time in physical activities.

  If you are not able to give up the news entirely, my recommendation is to only watch the newscast in the middle of the day (like the noon show or dinner time show). Some people watch the news several times a day. I feel the most harmful would be the shows immediately before bed or first thing in the morning.

Here I go again! My intention is not to put news people out of work, especially the late night teams. Even if this information reached, affected, and changed a million people, there would be several other millions to watch the news. My advice is only intended for people who are serious about Peace management. I can just envision the hate mail I will receive. Looks like I might need to practice Peace at a whole new level. Better yet, I hope the people tempted to send hate mail learn to practice Peace.

- I guess I also need to mention newspapers. You guessed it! I don't get the newspaper either. But please don't make me elaborate on this. I can't afford to alienate a whole new set of people. Figure this out on your own. But let me just share a headline I read on a table in a restaurant where we eat breakfast. It was in Cleveland's *Plain Dealer* on February 7, 2003. It read: "War Will Lead To Peace." Honest! Go figure!

  One student said "the only thing of value in the newspaper is the comics and the classified ads." He received a round of applause from the rest of the group. This makes me think that people understand the concept of toxicity from the media as a basic human instinct. If you surround yourself with stress, chaos, and fear, you will become a person who experiences stress, chaos, and fear.

- Exposure to people who are, for the most part, negative or who spend a great deal of time complaining could also be toxic to you. Watch your energy level after being around various people. After interactions with some people you may feel lighter or more joyful. After exposure to others, you may feel drained. Let those feelings be a guide for you, allowing yourself to remove whatever you feel is toxic.

- Analyze the things you find particularly toxic in your life. Some of my students comment about the stress or toxicity they feel in lines at stores. One student said she did not allow this silly thing to menace her. She does her grocery shopping at 11:00 pm. Another conversation spun off related to the stress and hostility that is felt in line at one local set of chain stores in particular. My students found it amusing when I pointed out to them that they are the only local chain stores that play the 24 hour, around-the-clock news on multiple TVs at the check out lines. We all got an ah-hah laugh at that one! Those poor cashiers. They are bombarded with news during their entire shift.

A side note: If you have to go shopping at a time when you know it will be crowded, just realize it is an opportunity to practice Peace. Believe it or not, sometimes I do this purposely. Just wait until the end of the book when I tell you what your final exam is!!!

Most of this section on toxicity relates back to the concept of valuing Peace and protecting it with every fiber of your body. At this point in your process, there is no better way to protect Peace than removing things you feel are toxic.

Remember, removing toxicity is only intended to be a temporary measure, while you are learning to be an effective Peace manager. By allowing yourself the space and time away from obvious, overt toxicity, you will move through the program and process quicker. I challenge you at some point, when you feel ready, to reintroduce the people you felt were toxic to your Peace back into your life. It will allow you to feel like you "made it." You then have the honor of wearing the graduation cap!

Exercise (N):

Remove Toxicity

Goals for this section:

- Identify the people or situations that you would label "toxic" to your Peace
- Consciously develop a plan for dealing with these toxicities

---

Activity A:

Make a list of the *people* you feel are currently toxic to your Peace

1. ______________________________

2. ______________________________

3. ______________________________

4. ______________________________

5. ______________________________

Did I give you enough lines?!?!?

If any of these people on your list live in the same house with you, make a commitment to move them to the top of your priority list, in terms of trying various techniques to achieve Peace in your interactions with them.

Activity B:

This one is not as hard. Make a list of *things* you find toxic to your Peace:

1. ______________________________

2. ______________________________

3. ______________________________

4. ______________________________

5. ______________________________

Make a plan for removing the toxicity from your existence, at least from the immediate future.

Activity C:

Make a plan for your eventual reintroduction of these people, and possibly, circumstances into your life.

Also, simultaneously, attempt to work on the technique of compassion, at least during your thoughts of the people you find toxic to your Peace.

Technique: Personality Self Analysis

Remember, I never said this was going to be easy. And this next technique may be one of the most difficult. It requires you to take a look at yourself, as you are your biggest asset and your own biggest detriment to experiencing life from a place of Peace.

I struggled with where to put this technique in the book. It really should be one of the earlier techniques, but you first need to see the value in the process before you are willing to look closely at yourself. Plus, there is an advantage in waiting a bit before introducing self analysis.

If you haven't already done so, you will soon become aware of a pattern to your growth process with Peace management, which is similar to any purposeful growth. You will witness a pattern of steps: tremendous growth, followed by a plateau, tremendous growth followed by another plateau, and so on. One strategy for taking growth to a new level is looking at the blocks to growth, followed by a willingness to remove them.

First, you need to see the value in growth before you will be willing to do the necessary work. How does continual growth relate to Peace? There seems to be a natural human instinct to continue to grow and evolve. It is unquestioned when related to the development of a baby or child. Somehow we lose the insight that growth is a continual process. Growth is human nature, stifled only when we resist it.

Therefore, when we stifle our human nature to evolve and grow, there is a subtle tugging and unrest in our spirit. The boredom and stagnation may be welcome on the surface, but to our essential selves, it is not desirable. This is often evident in a person soon after they retire. They welcome the idea of "having nothing to do." But very soon, their soul becomes agitated.

This came to light for me during a conversation with a former local political figure. I sat next to him at a dinner party. He poured his soul to me, telling me how he had anxiously awaited the slower pace of retirement. He had even sold his home and relocated to Florida, to have the ability to enjoy the weather and his activities year round. Well, you guessed it, he wound up with an extreme emptiness, a feeling that he lacked value. After having served such an important role in society for many years, settling into *just* being a "retired person" did not serve him well because he experienced stagnation and lack of challenge.

We spent a large part of our evening at that dinner party identifying the issues and then exploring ways to create areas of growth and challenge. I think you can easily see that, with stagnation, there could be a lack of Peace. So here is your challenge, which will serve as the platform for your continual personal growth . . . and be ready, I am going to shake you by your shackles again . . .

We all have personality traits that could directly interfere with Peace in a very obvious way. Below is a list of some of them, but these are not the ones I will be focusing on later:

- perfectionism
- procrastination
- impatience
- worrying about everything
- self pity
- need for control
- interference in other people's business
- rudeness
- self-defamation
- self-doubt
- self-centeredness
- victim mentality

It is important to look at these things and identify if any of them interfere with your Peace, how they interfere, and how to break past them. But there is another part of the self analysis that will be more personal, and harder to do. This is the analysis of the labels you apply to yourself. Before you read any further in this section, please turn to the following exercise (Exercise O) and complete activity A. It will be more helpful to you if you complete that section before being influenced by the content presented later in this section.

Often times we give labels to our attributes or traits as either a way to rationalize them or, worse yet, block growth or change in an area. Let's go to some examples. I may give myself the label of "good mother." This creates a subconscious resistance to any outside or internal challenge that I could be doing things differently or better. It lets me rest in this comfort zone. I do call myself a "good mother," but when I stop to be honest with myself, I soon realize there are several areas for potential improvement and growth. Labeling myself allows me to continue "as is." The lack of Peace comes in the resistance that I feel on some level, knowing I really could be better. And the resistance does not coincide with the words I use about myself.

Another example of a block to Peace, caused by blocking personal growth, relates to "positive" *adjectives* you might use to describe yourself. Let's say you describe yourself as "honest." Therefore, you won't acknowledge any activity you engage in that might represent a trifle lack of honesty. You might simply disregard the action as a fluke. This disregard doesn't allow you the opportunity to possibly choose differently, to align the behavior with your desired manifestation of your self.

Let's say you considered yourself honest. Your job is to market a new type of potato chip for a company. A store owner asks for your opinion of the potato chip. You happen not to care for the chip, but know there is a large market of people who do buy this product. You choose to answer by saying "it is a good potato chip." You feel you are being honest enough, because you side-stepped the question by not giving your personal opinion.

You knew the store owner was asking for your opinion, but you fail to acknowledge the lack of honesty in your answer, because you consider yourself to be honest. If you lost the label of "honest" as a description of yourself, you might actually answer with more honesty. You might have been able to say, "my taste in snack food is a little specific. I don't particularly care for it because I don't like salty foods. Therefore, my opinion of this potato chip is not relevant. But I do know there is a large segment of the population who thinks this product is good, because we sell a lot of it." Do you see that by not allowing yourself to hide behind the label of honest, you could be more free to answer from your heart?

On the opposite end, if you give yourself a "negative" label, this allows you to rationalize lack of growth. If you say, "I am unorganized," this allows you the freedom from the effort it takes to become more organized. If you say, "I am forgetful," it takes the burden off you to try to be more attentive to things. Did you notice that the "negative" words were fairly acceptable socially? Look closer. Could these "negative" labels actually be blocking you from using less socially-acceptable labels? Is it better for you to say "I am unorganized or forgetful" than to say "I am lazy"? Are you getting to see how this labeling really blocks self knowledge and growth thereby limiting our Peace?

When I was in nursing administration, one of our supervisors openly called herself "unorganized." She did have several other assets and did contribute a great deal to the team. However, her repeated organizational failures, in addition to the fact the she frequently called herself "unorganized" excused her from certain responsibilities. This created a larger burden on the rest of us. When a project was needed and it was time to divide up the work, my director would actually say things like "let's not have Amy write the policy and procedures (sometimes even with a chuckle that had us all chuckle); we'll just have her at the meeting to help us sell the idea." That meant that the rest of us had to divide up the tedious, burdensome work while Amy graciously was excused from the work. She may or may not have seen this as an escape from work, but it definitely blocked her growth, because it was acceptable to have this label.

Let's move to a slightly different type of labeling. It is the type of labeling that *makes me right*. The best example is the way people apply the concepts of optimism and pessimism. I believe that optimism and pessimism exist on a continuum, all the way from very optimistic to very pessimistic. Have you ever noticed that everyone who falls from the mid point of the continuum, all the way to the extreme point on the pessimistic side of the continuum, always refers to themselves as a realist, while no one on the optimistic half of the continuum calls themselves a realist? Let's look at this.

"Pessimist" as a label, is not particularly favorable. "Realist" would be a more favorable word. It is more self-preserving to think of yourself in a positive way (even for a pessimist). Therefore, it is the rationalization for having a certain perspective on life.

Let's look at how foolish it is to have a label as a "realist" in the first place. We are talking about perception, not fact. So how can perception be real? It is not fact. Let's say we are evaluating the work of a carpenter. The pessimist might think it is a terrible job, the optimist might think it is a great job. They are both using their own set of criteria to judge the situation. Is one person's set of criteria more real?

Take that to world affairs. One person might think things in the world are getting better, another might think they are getting worse. The one who thinks things are getting worse would be on the pessimistic side of the continuum. But to allow their train of thinking to prevail, they call themselves a realist.

If the optimist thinks their perception is the accurate one, they might also be blocking growth. They may not being open to the possibility there is another way to look at things. Not being open to variations of opinion keeps us in a very limited box.

Well, how do we change this? Don't give yourself a label. Rather than telling myself, "I am a good mother," I can think myself as "*practicing* being a good mother." You obviously don't have to say this out loud (you would sound kind of silly), but just allow it to be the way you think. On a subconscious level, this gives me permission to keep working on something that is desirable to me. If you don't have the mentality of practicing, you will think of a character trait as an absolute and defend any need to consider changing or growing.

Sometimes labels are necessary, for example, at work when describing your role. It is helpful for my colleagues and patients to know I am a nurse. But during the rest of life, it is not helpful to allow the label of your role to interfere with the way you experience life. For example, if I allowed the label "I am a mom" to interfere with life, I might not snow board with my son or read Harry Potter. I really want to try those things and if I hid behind my role, I might make other choices. I would be at a lack of Peace on a subtle level, because I am not being true to myself.

Another aspect of personality analysis is looking at things you believe serve you fairly well, but are not inherently desirable to you. An example came to light with a couple I worked with. They were both nurses. The husband was very controlling in his relationship with his wife. A small group of his nursing colleagues brought this controlling nature to his attention. He acknowledged it, but simply said "it's just the way I am. Things are fine." But we sensed he did not really like being that way because we felt the unrest in his spirit when he acted in a controlling way.

Well things may have been "fine" for a while, but this man's wife eventually left him. Her reason: he was too controlling. He thought that by controlling his wife and the situation, he could keep their comfort and their life at the status quo. It worked for a while, but things that are not based on honesty with your desired self are eventually a breeding ground for upheaval. Not only did the husband feel bad in the controlling role, but the wife experienced a resentment in allowing herself to succumb to his control, knowing she deeply wished for a different way. The concept of acting in a way that is authentic and true to yourself will be looked at again in "Peace from Total Integrity."

Before we move on, I would like to bring your attention to another related concept: the use of words. Words, in general, block growth in abstract areas. Words are symbols of symbols (twice removed). For example, "chair" is the *word symbol* for that thing, that is a *function symbol* for a piece of furniture that is used for sitting. And "chair" is a concrete concept. Think about our use of the words "love" or "apathy". Image the benefit in evolving as a person (not in everyday functions) if human beings were deaf and mute, and had no ability to communicate in writing. We would only be able to communicate with energy, mood, and expression. This would allow us to focus on experiencing. Imagine life without words. See what this thought does to you.

Hospitals, doctors, and nurses are finally realizing that words are what get them in trouble with lawyers. The words in the charts are what lawyers try to interpret in a manipulative way for monetary benefit. (and "no" I have never been involved in a law suit, not even deposed, thank God). Hospitals are finally changing charting to minimal necessary wording. This comes from years of learning the hard way.

The use of words falls short in attempting to communicate. But they are the best we have. Imagine a hospital where, if someone was sick they would just come into the hospital, and we would take care of them. Yes, I know this is a ridiculous concept. We do need words, but it certainly makes you realize how we can be hung by our words and how we incompletely communicate through use of words. This also happens in day-to-day conversations with people. We do need words, carefully chosen words, to communicate with others and to understand ourselves better. But remember the use of words has limitations. Be careful in your choice of words at all times, because they are not only used in attempting to communicate, but they also create you and the perpetuation of your thoughts.

Remember, our goal is to continually take Peace to a higher and higher level. Not only will Peace influence the things that you do and the way that you are, but it will totally change your energy. You don't want things to hold you back or hold you down. I'd like to give you a visual to help guide your progress: Which do you think is more in line with the vibrational frequency of light: a slug or a garden fairy? What is your energy goal?

<u>Exercise (O)</u>:

Personality Self Analysis

Goals for this section:

- Identify the labels and adjectives you use to describe yourself
- Determine if your labels and self-descriptions block your growth
- Explore your ideas on how the use of words may inhibit your growth

---

<u>Activity A:</u>

Take a moment to write down all the labels you have for your roles (dad, lawyer, son, committee chair, speaker for men's health group)

Write down the "positive" words that you use to describe yourself. They should be adjectives (loyal, kind, attentive, courageous)

Write down the "negative" words that you use to describe yourself. They should also be adjectives (forgetful, slow, too focused, too anything)

Activity B:

Take a moment to analyze the growth that may be blocked by your labels. For example, if you say "I am a good teacher," are you blocking creativity that would allow you to be a better teacher?

Determine if any of the "negative" adjectives you use to describe yourself rationalize or allow stagnation in an area. For example, if you say "I am just a worrier", does that give you the permission to obsessively ask questions of other people (kids, spouse, co-workers)?

Activity C:

This is a fun experiment. Try not saying very much today. Try communicating without too many words. Watch the responses in other people.

Also, in your imagination, play out how your work setting and home setting might improve if no one talked.

Activity D:

Determine if any of the "seriousness" of your roles blocks you from engaging in activities that would promote any type of growth or enjoyment. For example, "I am a secretary in the payroll department and could never take off on a Tuesday." Did you miss your child's Christmas concert because of the restrictions you place on yourself with your role? Could you have been creative in finding a way to meet your responsibilities at work and attend the concert?

Remember, I am a mom (in my mid 40s), but I had a blast snow boarding!

Activity E:

This activity is intended to expand your thinking. What do you think someone might be blocking if they use these phrases?

- I am not confrontational
- I am too old
- I have great self esteem
- I have become apathetic
- I don't have enough time
- I can't afford it
- I do best with a deadline
- I don't care
- I don't like to give or get presents
- I am too busy
- I am not athletic enough
- I date the wrong type of men/women

The list could go on and on . . .

Technique: Promote peace

After working through the heavy topics, "removing toxicity" and "personality self analysis," covering a more up beat topic will be a nice change of pace. This section will focus on identifying and implementing strategies to create the opportunity for you to have more Peace in your life by promoting peace, enjoyment, and relaxation.

These techniques that enhance your external world to promote calmness are by no means intended to replace the transformation that leads to inner Peace. They can evolve simultaneously. However, the process cannot work in reverse. You cannot approach changing your environment or external circumstances with the hope that this will create the inner Peace you desire.

One student said "I will have more Peace when I am finished with school." Her life may be more calm, but she will not have more Peace unless she chooses it. And she can choose it now, while she is in school.

Similarly, I recently moved from a busy suburb to the country. If I had thought moving to the country would bring me Peace, I would have been in for a big disappointment. Luckily, I was already a Peace manager, so moving to the country just represented more calm in my life. With this awareness, I didn't have the unrealistic expectations that many have about the benefits of moving to the country.

The techniques of promoting peace will be presented in two categories. The first focuses on pleasures of the senses. The second focuses on lifestyle practices. Some of you may initially think this information is not as valuable as the meatier topics, but this section is not that long. Even if you come away with one tip to create a more peaceful environment or more easily flowing lifestyle it will be worth it. The few minutes to read this section may provide some real benefit for you.

First let's start by promoting pleasure of the senses. As an educator, I know and accommodate the fact that different senses are dominant in different people. Actually, educators incorporate the concept of "taking in" and learning via multiple senses. Multiple senses also play a role in situations other than learning. For instance, you experience life through your interpretation of sensory input and information. Knowing this, you may decide to pay more attention to one or more of your senses.

Sound

Let's start with the *auditory sense*. Obviously, quiet is good, but I would like to focus on sounds that are pleasing and therefore, peaceful for you. Here are some suggestions:

- The sound of running water is peaceful. I have incorporated the peaceful sound of water into my life in a variety of ways. I have a water fountain at work, two at home, and a small waterfall in my back yard. I have a meditation garden by a running stream. My jogging course leads past a very active waterfall. I make certain I leave enough time to just sit and listen to the running water.

- Any continuous sound is peaceful. Examples are
    - fire (like a fireplace or a bonfire)
    - wind (go sit outside on a windy day)
    - rain (especially if you can sit in a place where you hear it on a roof)
    - a clock that you can hear ticking

- Music that you find calming. Different music works well for different people. There are specific record companies that cater to this need. You can purchase CDs with nature sounds, instrumentals, classical music, bells, chants, or one of a variety of other sound techniques that are aimed at promoting peacefulness.

- Sometimes sounds are utilized to initiate meditation. I have a crystal bowl that when rubbed emits a continuous bell-type sound that allows me to focus. You can experiment with other sound techniques to help you enter meditation (or stillness of the mind).

- Avoid exposure to unpleasant sounds. I am on the zoning board of appeals in my town. We just concluded an appeal process where residents bordering a sand and gravel plant complained about the loud and obnoxious sounds they are forced to deal with, coupled with the low-level continuous sounds. My heart went out to them. Most lived there before the plant began operating. These people were out of luck, but the potential for noise in a neighborhood should be taken into consideration when deciding where you will live and spend your "quiet time". Avoid any other unpleasant noises when you are trying to promote a life that is peaceful.

Sight

Now let's tackle *visual*. There are a variety of modifications you can implement to make your environment more pleasing to the eye and therefore, more peaceful:

- My first suggestion is to de-clutter. If you have clutter in your environment, you can have a lack of ease inside of you, weighing you down. Utilize whatever techniques are suited for your personal situation to get the mess at least out of sight. Of course, it would be best not to hide the clutter, but to actually get rid of it.

  I realize that when you marry someone, you should not try to change them or their ways. But I needed to confront something before I married my husband. Basically, I needed to know if he would allow me to manage the papers and bookkeeping in our marriage. His style would have created a very unpeaceful (is that a word?) environment for me. Luckily, my husband obliged. He was very neat and clean, but had multiple piles of papers in *every* room (yes, even the bathroom, bedrooms, and dining room). I have to admit, he could find most things he needed, but it would have made me feel very unsettled.

How do you handle the paper mess? Three ring notebooks and file cabinets are great inventions. In my home, if it doesn't belong in a notebook or a file cabinet, it belongs in the garbage!

How do you handle the other clutter? Allow yourself one junk drawer in each room. And that's it. If it doesn't fit in the drawer, time to start purging. All "junk" and trinkets should be out of sight.

- Pay special attention to the entrance of your home. If you tend to come in through the garage, de-clutter and clean this area and the first room where you enter the house. It sets the tone for your experience of being at home. Don't allow yourself to fall in the rut of putting things on the washer/dryer, for example if that is the first flat surface you encounter in your home.

- Pay attention to the lighting in your home. In some areas you will probably want bright light, in other areas you might want soft lighting. Try candles for dinner. Try candles everywhere. Candles create a relaxing atmosphere.

- You might want to research Feng Shui. I don't have much personal experience regarding this oriental environment planning technique, but many of my students use this concept as a framework for projects. For example, I had one group of students use Feng Shui to design a hospital room that promoted peace. I liked what I saw!

- In decorating, use colors that are pleasing to you and peaceful in nature. Experiment with this. I suggest trying muted or pastel colors.

Smell

Now the *olfactory sense*. Here are some ideas for promoting peace through your nose. This is a big one for me. I often joke, "if there is a hell, mine will be one where there are horrible smells." I just want to "toss my cookies" when I enter a house where there is a combination of an old dog and old carpeting. I actually gave up a stint of home nursing because of this specific type of odor.

One fourth of July, I was assigned a patient who had just been discharged from the hospital, and she had a new tracheostomy tube (hole in her neck attached to a breathing machine). I was at her home for an eight hour shift. That shift felt like it lasted 48 hours. It was a lovely family, but they had three ancient dogs and 30 year old carpeting. That carpeting had the memory of everything it had ever been exposed to. That was my last full shift in home nursing. I would only agree to brief visits after that.

Think of your own home or work environment. Are there any noxious or unpleasant smells to which you are exposed? Where do you keep your trash can? Do you clean out your indoor waste baskets regularly? Do your pets need any hygiene help? Do you or any of your family members need any hygiene help? Be kind, but be honest with them.

Every time I go on vacation, I get a new perfume or lotion. Therefore, if I ever need a little pick-me-up from dull routine at home, I put on a little perfume, and I am transported back to a peaceful beach or an exciting city.

You may also want to try using scents throughout the house: air fresheners, scented candles, scented oils, or lamp rings. I use various types of incense to create different feelings. They are fun to experiment with.

Taste

Now, the *gustatory sense*. Probably my favorite one to indulge. Go ahead, please your taste buds! (Now I am not talking about taking it to the point of gluttony.) Taste is probably more individualized than the other senses. Figure out your favorites (if you haven't already), and experience the pleasure of satisfying your gustatory sense. On occasion, I have been know to have very taste-pleasing meals (with minimal nutritional value), simply for the gustatory pleasure. I am an adult. If I want lime flavored chips for dinner, I will have lime flavored chips for dinner!

Touch

Tactile - the sense of feel or touch. I have a few suggestions:

- Wear clothes that feel good on your skin, especially if you are going to be in them for several hours.

- Don't wear anything that is constricting, tight, or rides up. Yuk! There is not much that will distract me more than uncomfortable clothing. It saddens me to admit that I am at a point in my life where comfort matters, but it does. When you buy a new pair of shoes, break them in slowly, and take a spare pair of comfortable shoes with you, in case you need a change. Don't depend on wearing your new shoes your entire work day or formal occasion. It is smart to keep an extra pair of shoes in the car.

- Forget the heavy earrings, or only wear them for brief periods of time.

- Don't wear uncomfortable pajamas (nothing that gets twisted, will cause you to get too warm or cold, or is too tight).

- I highly recommend treating yourself to a massage occasionally. They are therapeutic on many levels. I got hooked early in life, when I owned a health spa. I don't spend money on my hair and nails, so it is easy for me to rationalize the cost of this indulgence. It is a wonderful tactile experience.

Multi-sensual

Before we move on to the second category, here are a few ideas for creating pleasant environments using multiple senses:

- Make all your spaces pleasing and comfortable for you. If you have an office in your work setting, you might want to de-institutionalize it. I don't think I could be relaxed or creative in an institutional beige office. My office at the college has pleasing colors, dresser scarves, plants, a fountain, a CD player for peaceful music, and soft lighting.

- I encourage everyone to have a "sacred space" in their home; one where you feel comfortable even if the rest of the house is in desperate need of attention. It could be as simple as a chair with an end table next to it that has a candle, a good thought-provoking book, a dish of scented oils, and, of course, chocolate.

- Locate a place outdoors that is "your space." Even if it is not really your space or where you live. It could be a special place in a park, near a river, under a certain tree, anyplace where you can go to regroup and reenergize. Don't ever use that place to take someone else in order to "work out" a problem. You want it to be a place that you associate with pleasant experiences.

- Pay close attention to your bedroom. It is the first place you see in the morning and the last place you see at night. Have essentials in reach on your night stand (some suggestions: a glass of water, a notebook and pen, tissues, a good reading lamp, and your Peace management book).

The second main category of peace promotion deals with lifestyle issues. I think the most important issue in promoting peace is time management. Not that we can manage time. It has a mind of its own, but we can determine how we use this wonderful resource. I strongly emphasize this with my nursing students. It is an absolute must for success in nursing. Nurses, like many other professionals, have to continually prioritize and reprioritize and reprioritize. If they don't, they will sink.

Nurses, especially in ER or other critical care settings, use the concept of triage. This concept can be applied to many aspects of life. Essentially, it is the practice of revolving priorities. You continually take into account new concerns and all former concerns and decide what gets your attention now. When you get comfortable with this concept, it relieves you of the burden of feeling that you have to do everything now. We all have only have one now. And the whole multi-tasking concept has added an additional feeling of burden. Multi-tasking is only beneficial up to a point and only in certain circumstances. We need to be conscious of our own limits and the diminishing returns on effort spread too thinly.

The benefit of time management, in general (besides getting things done), is that you will have plenty of time to play and relax. I manage many activities, but I would never fill up my schedule to the point where I would compromise my fun or my relaxing time. I value them too much!

You must also pay attention to how much sleep you need. Figure out how long you sleep when you are not wakened by an alarm. Watch this over time. Then make getting this amount of sleep that your body wants your goal. Protect your sleep. In the past, I wanted to go for the jugular of people who said "I only need five hours of sleep each night." (This was obviously before I became a Peace manager.) I knew I needed more than five hours. I finally figured out I need nine hours of sleep a night. Now I protect that time intensely. I function at a much higher level when I have the right amount of sleep.

One other related point: I think it is very difficult to be a successful Peace manager when your physiological needs are not met. I agree with Maslow. We need to take care of our basic human survival needs before we can begin to think about any higher level needs. You cannot be hungry, exhausted, thirsty, or gasping for air and work on Peace management.

Here are some other things to consider when you are attempting to make your external world and lifestyle more peaceful:

- spend time outdoors
- regularly meditate (quiet your mind)
- regularly exercise (or at least be active)
- use relaxation techniques when needed
- embrace change
- go to bed ½ hour early and wake up ½ hour early
- don't procrastinate (You will eventually get to the point, as a Peace manager where you could wait until April 14th to do your taxes, but wonder why people do that.)
- follow the old saying: when life gives you lemons, make lemonade
- don't over spend
- be around fresh flowers or plants
- get a handle on your finances
- spend time with old people or children (unless this makes you nuts)
- volunteer for anything you feel is worthwhile
- schedule time with friends
- find a creative outlet
- treat yourself as well as you would a neighbor
- move toward regularly feeling gratitude and appreciation

Have fun evaluating your environment with open eyes (and ears, nose, skin, and tongue). Gradually make changes until your environment reflects who you are and adds to the peace in your life. Enjoy the creative process.

<u>Exercise (P)</u>:

Promote peace

Goals for this section:

- Identify areas in your environment that could be altered to promote peace
- Focus on improving your external environment by paying attention to each of the five senses
- Identify lifestyle modifications which would allow you to incorporate more peace in your life

---

<u>Activity A:</u>

List "problem areas" you currently identify in your environment that lack a sense of peace.

<u>Activity B:</u>

How could you make your environment more pleasing to the eye?

How could you make your environment more pleasing to the ear?

How could you make your environment more pleasing to the nose?

How could you make your environment more pleasing to the skin?

How could you make your environment more pleasing to the taste buds?

Activity C:

Analyze your current life. Identify the current chaos and stressors. Make a plan to reasonably modify these external stressors.

Technique: Still Your Mind

With your exposure to the earlier techniques, your practice with the advancing techniques, and a general appreciation of Peace, you are probably becoming aware that your mind goes non-stop!!! As you progress through the process, you become more acutely aware of this non-stop activity. Your mind judges, thinks of the past, creates fears and anguish about the future, engages in thoughts that cause suffering, races to thoughts that cause an emotion or charge, plus the endless day-to-day types of thoughts, like your grocery list, who is picking up the kids tonight, which library books need to get back, and on, and on, and on . . .

Therefore, it is time to work on stilling you mind. In addition to practicing specific techniques to manage your Peace, you need simultaneously to practice techniques to still your mind. There is no way to truly achieve Peace during the constant monkey chatter going on in your mind. In a sense, you need to prove to yourself that you are the master of your mind and your mind is not the master of you.

I have been utilizing many mind stilling techniques over the years, even before Peace management came into existence. One of the periods in my life when I gained the most appreciation for stilling the mind was in 2003, when I was participating in a study group. It was hosted in my home and facilitated by a man I respect beyond description. He is a friend and long time student of "A Course in Miracles." Plus, he is well versed in many other teachings. Because I always look to him for advice on areas for my development, I affectionately refer to him as "Swami J." He understands things on such a deep level and strongly advocates stilling the mind. He led the group to actualizing the techniques to effectively still our minds.

The study group discussed the book *The Power of Now* by Eckhart Tolle. Three techniques that we practiced in the study group are as follows:

1. When you cannot still your mind, when the thoughts are just racing through you head, stop and ask yourself "What will my next thought be?"

   This question causes your mind to be still, if only for a moment. This anticipation or waiting allows you to be in a state that is absent of thought. It gives you a taste of having a still mind. This exercise is one of the most helpful in teaching the concept of a still mind to my students.

2. Practice being in the Moment, or as Tolle calls it "in the Now." Some suggestions for practice are: when you are walking in to work, notice the temperature of the air, the landscaping, or the weight of your purse or briefcase. Or when you are eating, feel the texture of the food and the variations of taste as the food moves around your mouth.

3. When you are looking at things, take the focus off the things and allow your attention to fall between the things. For example, look between the trees or between the cups, but not at what makes the backdrop behind the items, simply the space in between.

Any one of these or other techniques that takes your mind out of the mode of constant processing will aid in your gradual ability to still your mind.

I would now like to suggest several other techniques to promote stillness of the mind:

- Turn off your car radio when you are in the car by yourself. It may not seem like it interferes with stillness, but it is a constant, close bombardment of noise. It keeps your brain engaged, even if you don't think you are really listening. Plus, this time is a great opportunity to practice several of the other techniques in this program. I am not suggesting that you drive in silence all the time. I don't want any nasty letters from radio DJs. I am just suggesting you occasionally try silence as a way to include mind stillness in your day.

- Consciously focus on your breathing. It is something that you can do anytime, anyplace. The rhythmic nature and continual nature of breathing provide a great focus for your attention. When I say focus upon it, I mean *only* it. Do not allow your concentration to wander. And if it does, bring your attention right back to your breath.

- While you are walking, be aware of each time your foot meets the ground. Allow your awareness to rest there.

- Light a candle and focus on the flame. Any focused concentration will at least temporarily still the mind.

- A very helpful technique in promoting discipline of your mind is something I refer to as *fizzle the thought*. It takes great dedication, desire, and discipline to have a still mind. It is a gradual process. Therefore, an early technique that can be used as a form of discipline is becoming aware of the constant thought stream. Once the awareness is present, fizzle the current thought you are having. You will experience a momentary stillness of your mind. When another thought enters, fizzle it immediately. You can use a form of imagery to assist with the process. You can either imagine that your thought is a stick of firmly packed powder, that disintegrates into fine powder and blows away as the thought fizzles or you can imagine it as a lighted fuse of a fire cracker. The burning spark on the fuse fizzles out before it detonates the explosive, just as the thought burns out into *no thought*.

Begin developing your own individualized techniques for having at least momentary stillness of the mind. The more skilled you become, the longer the periods of stillness will endure.

Peace is our natural state, and you will eventually see Peace and stillness as effortless. *Knowing* about Peace will not get you there. *You must experience it*. When your mind is still, there is no room for stress, fear, or anger. Mastering stillness will take you one step closer to the ability to experience Peace on a more regular basis.

Relaxation is a co-requisite for stillness. There are many relaxation techniques you can utilize to approach stillness and Peace. I don't advocate any particular path. They all work to accomplish the same end. You can get tapes, videos, and books from the library. Or you can rely on whatever has successfully allowed you to enter a relaxed feeling in the past. Relaxation helps stillness; stillness helps relaxation. Please make note that there is a significant difference between simple relaxation and stillness.

Meditation is a deeper experience of stillness. Meditation is something I practice throughout the day, spontaneously, as well as during designated times. The benefit of the stillness and Peace is indescribable.

Meditation, like relaxation techniques, can be practiced in a variety of different ways. I have tried many different techniques. It is not important which approach you take as long as you sit quietly, in a passive state, with the intention of experiencing no mental or physical activity. In the beginning, most individuals need a specific technique to get themselves to shut down and allow a state of meditative awareness to occur.

Like I said, I have tried a variety of techniques. If you would like to research some of these techniques, you can search for information on the use of mantras, sound, breathing techniques, visual focus, imagery, music, or bells. Most of the time, I can go into a meditative state instantly. I don't know if that ability came out of necessity, due to time constraints, or if it is because once one experiences a meditative state it is easy to call back.

If you don't have time to research meditation, I have provided two examples of imagery that you can use to still your mind, to promote entry into a meditative state. These two imagery techniques are presented in the exercise following this technique section.

No matter what techniques you use to still your mind, you will immediately reap the benefit of experiencing temporary freedom from a runaway mind. Enjoy!

Exercise (Q):

Still Your Mind

Goals for this section:

- Practice the techniques presented to still your mind
- Develop your own techniques to experience stilling of your mind
- Practice meditation

Activity A:

Go back to the text section of the book for a description of each of these techniques. Practice each one of the following techniques, some time during the next week:

- Ask yourself "what is my next thought?" and watch what happens.

- Pay special attention to your surroundings as you enter work tomorrow. Notice everything, but do not attach any judgment or meaning to anything.

- Sit down by yourself and eat something. Become acutely aware of the texture and flavor of the food. Become aware of the swallowing of the food. Do not let any thought enter your mind during this experience.

- Look in between objects to see the space.

- Turn off the car radio. Become aware of the absence of noise.

- Take time to focus your awareness only on your breathing.
- While you are walking, focus only on your foot meeting the ground.
- Light a candle and focus only on the flame. Do not let any thought enter that time.

Activity B:

Develop your own techniques to still your mind, and write down what they are for future reference:

-
-
-
-
-

Activity C:

Practice meditation. Attempt to utilize each of these imagery techniques to start off your meditation period.

First, get yourself into a comfortably seated position with your back straight, if possible. Support your body in a very relaxed manner. Allow your muscles to relax, including the muscles in your face. Close your eyes and focus on your breathing for a few cycles, allowing nothing else to enter your mind. The two imagery exercises I have developed allow you to still your mind without feeling a need to punish yourself when your mind breaks the stillness with some random thoughts. Random thoughts will intrude a great deal, especially at first.

Note: it helps me during my pre-meditative state, not to do a visual imagery. The visual image is actually distracting to me. When I refer to "your mind's eye," I mean a feeling rather than a visual picture of something.

- Imagine, in your minds eye, a flowing river, running right past you. When you get to a very relaxed state with your mind becoming still, imagine that the river stops and expands out into a motionless pond of water, right in front of you. As long as you are in the relaxed state with a still mind, keep feeling the still pond. As soon as a thought comes into your mind, allow the river to begin moving again and carry that thought with it down river. Once the thought is gone, focus upstream again, at the moving river. When you are relaxed again with a still mind, allow the river to become still again, creating a large still pond in front of you. Continue this process as each new thought enters until you are done with your session.

- The closest we can get to experiencing eternity or Peace is in the Now or the current Moment. During this meditation, once your eyes are closed, experience the Now. It gradually becomes an ever-expanding now, expanding in all directions and in all dimensions. It is all-encompassing. As soon as a thought enters your mind, come right back to a very small image of Now, allowing it to re-expand as you relax again to that total encompassing Now. Repeat this as needed during your session of meditation.

Technique: Don't Go There

This technique builds on "Remove Toxicity." It is the technique that is used when a situation that could be distressing is occuring. You simply say to yourself "don't go there" or you could say to another person "I am not going there." My husband gets what this is about and we stop our discussion immediately. My son may challenge me a bit, until he realizes that I really am "not going there" and he realizes all his efforts will be wasted.

For example, I am not thrilled about driving in snow, but my husband is not bothered by snow or rain conditions during driving. One day, my husband and I were shuttling two cars to a lot. The roads were heavily snow covered. In a very matter-of-fact way, he began telling me how pulling his trailer behind his van helped him get better traction in the snow, but it also made stopping more challenging. He also started telling me about a couple of close-calls he had while navigating the hills on his way in to work. I just stopped him dead in his tracks. The thought of him on hills in the snow, or the possibility of difficulty with stopping a vehicle was overwhelming. I was tired and hungry, and I did not have the energy to resist stress and maintain Peace. I knew that if the conversation about the dangers of driving in snow continued (especially while we were driving on snow covered roads), I wouldn't be able to hold back stress and maintain my Peace. I said "I don't want to feel stress, so I don't want to discuss this any more right now." My husband easily obliged because he understands Peace management. In other words, I said "don't go there".

Another obvious time to use this technique is when you feel someone is trying to pull you into a drama where you don't belong. You can say "I know this issue is important to you, but I don't feel I should be involved." Again, in other words you are saying "I'm not going there."

There are many other situations that would warrant this technique. I encounter many such situations. Someone new to my life was very controlling in nature. I could easily have been drawn into the drama that plays out when you try to resist being controlled. You know how that scene goes. You might give all kinds of reasons why you don't want to take their "suggestion", (why am I being so kind? - their "demand") or you may act in a passive-aggressive way (agree with them to their face, but then do the complete opposite). Neither choice feels good. Both can bring on a charge. Therefore, I scripted a line that I used every time this particular individual began "suggesting." I would say "I will take that into consideration when I am making my decision." It stopped the conversation immediately. There was nothing else to be said. Neither one of us had a charge. And basically, I was saying "I am not going there."

One friend used a great variation of this technique. She was involved in a custody case that was in active legal negotiations. She received a letter from her attorney on a Saturday. Rather than open the letter, read its contents, and have the possible bad news on her mind all weekend, she decided to put it aside until Monday. She knew she would not be able to reach her attorney over the weekend anyway, and she didn't want to ruin the fun weekend she had planned with her kids. We joked and imagined it was simply a thank you card from her attorney, for paying his last month's Jaguar payment. My friend decided "not to go there."

I have slight hypoglycemia (low blood sugar). It is manifested by my feeling irritable. When I know I am in need of protein and someone tries to engage me in conversation, I say "we better talk about this later." I am not in the frame of mind or mood to talk. I simply "don't go there."

Don't react to statements when other people share their opinions of you. This could trigger one of your "buttons." There is a great saying: *it is none of my business what other people think of me.* Don't be pulled in. Don't go there.

Identify what your buttons are. What are those statements and situations that make the hair on the back on your neck stand on end? Know your buttons and why they are buttons. This way, when others try to push those buttons in an attempt to weaken you or manipulate you, you are on to their strategy, so it cannot work for them. You will be less tempted to "go there" when you know the other person is trying to manipulate, control, or weaken you.

Realize they are only *your* buttons. If someone said the same words to me that they said to you, I might not react because they don't affect me. They are not *my* buttons. For example, if someone made a snide comment about me not carrying my weight on a project, it wouldn't affect me. I don't have that image of myself. Yet if something inside you makes you feel like you don't always give 100%, you may be very sensitive to those type of comments. You need to figure out why your buttons are your buttons. Once you know them, when someone else tries to use them, don't go there.

Don't take on negative emotions of others. Make it a conscious choice. I went to hear a motivational speaker. The audience was energized, yet calm. However, when the speaker started making a point by using stories from current events that were tragic and scary, I noticed a shift in the mood of the whole audience. There was a restlessness. The restlessness grew stronger as time went on because people started picking up the restless energy from the people sitting next to them.

I recognized the discomfort in the room and went into my "don't go there" mode. I didn't want to shift out of the positive emotions I had been feeling earlier, and I am very aware of the power of group consciousness. Finally, the mood broke and the calm returned. We must realize that we can be pulled from our Peace into negativity and become a part of a group energy. That is okay if it is a positive emotion, but don't get sucked into something that you do not want to experience. Don't go there.

This may seem painfully obvious, but I can't tell you how many people don't get this. Don't commit crimes! Being married to a sergeant of a detective bureau, I can't help but think about this. If people stopped for a moment to think about the consequences of their actions before engaging in criminal activity, they could spare themselves the embarrassment, the expense, and yes, the stress of being arrested. Even something that they may consider a "minor annoyance" could actually create their entry into the criminal justice system. Don't go there!

My son has "current events" in school. Last night, in his backpack was the *News Herald* from March 16, 2004. There was a big picture of Martha Stewart, with a caption that read: "Martha Stewart . . . handed over her keys to the executive suite of the media empire she built, Monday, a little more than a week after she was convicted on four federal charges." I don't know any of the specifics of this case, but I can't help but think that she was probably not in a place of Peace at that moment.

Some violations that may seem relatively benign can make you need to talk to the police, and possibly enter a distressing arena are:

- ◊ harassing phone calls
- ◊ trespassing
- ◊ pranks that end up damaging property
- ◊ retribution of an ex-spouse or employer
- ◊ stalking (a pattern of following or harassing)
- ◊ writing a bad check when you don't have sufficient funds
- ◊ violating building or zoning codes

There are several other "minor" crimes that become major ordeals when the person being victimized decides to press charges.

Hopefully, I have made the point that it is easier to choose not to "go there" than to deal with the external and the internal consequences.

Exercise (R):

Don't Go There

Goals for this section:

- *Prevent* situations which would normally produce a charge for you
- Identify your "buttons" and analyze the reason they are "buttons"
- Create an awareness that it is your choice to avoid stressful situations

---

Activity A:

Think of recent situations or conversations that created a charge. Could this technique have been used to prevent entry into the situation?

Develop a plan to utilize should a similar situation arise. If it is a situation that seems to repeat itself, consider scripting a line you could use that would be effective and kind.

Activity B:

Identify your specific "buttons." You will know they are your buttons by the way you feel and the way you react. It may help to look at conversations you have with people close to you. Believe me, they know your buttons. They may have no malicious intent, but simply, have learned how to get what they want.

Think about the origin of your buttons. Why do you react so strongly when those particular buttons are pushed? This may actually help you analyze things about your personality that block your growth.

Make a plan not to "go there" when you become aware that someone is trying to "push your buttons."

Technique: Go There

The "go there" technique nicely follows the discussion of having your "buttons" pushed. "Go there" gives you more insight and a specific technique when someone is trying to push your buttons. However, this technique has broader application than simply a strategy to use when someone pushes your buttons. This technique encourages you to "go there" to places that may not be very comfortable initially, but will assist you in your practice of Peace.

For example, when you feel a resistance to something or find yourself strongly defending something, this technique will work well. I use it often. When you feel yourself wanting to resist or defend, you need to examine what it is that you are fighting so hard *not* to feel. This awareness is the first step. When this awareness comes to me, I actually go and isolate myself for a bit, to try to figure out what I'm reacting to.

Let's apply "go there" to some real life situations. Let's say your wife says "did you *remember* to pick up the milk on your way home?" And the way she emphasizes "remember", triggers an emotional response. A "no" might be sufficient, yet you feel like you want to defend yourself. You might begin with all kinds of excuses, rationalizations, or even lash out at your wife. When you look closer, you may be acting in a way designed to protect yourself from feeling a certain way about yourself. You may be trying to resist feeling like you are irresponsible, forgetful, or any other negative label you can think of. But for the sake of this example, let's say you are trying to resist feeling irresponsible.

At this point in the process, I have to *physically* isolate myself because the issues are often more complex than I can handle in a flash thought. I usually excuse myself and say "I will be back in a bit." Taking a time out to gather your thoughts is part of the first step. Let's say the husband above takes this advice and goes to isolate himself. When he figures out that he is resisting feeling irresponsible, he has entered the second step. He knows that if he doesn't do some work here, the conversation will take its typical path, where his wife tries to help him be more responsible and he defends his actions in an attempt not to feel irresponsible.

Next is the work. What the husband needs to do is, in a quiet environment, close his eyes, and actually feel what it is he is trying to resist feeling. He should feel what it feels like to "feel irresponsible." (Go ahead, read that sentence again). He needs to take some time and completely feel it. Suddenly, he will realize that the feeling was not as bad as he thought it would be. Feeling irresponsible is not the end of the world. Life does not cease to exist. The husband will realize that there is nothing more his wife can do to him that he hasn't already done to himself.

This recognition places the husband in a frame of mind to be more open to hearing what his wife has to say. He does not have to agree with her, but at least he is not defending himself, which prevents him from really hearing her perspective. He can continue the conversation without a charge.

To take another example, let's say your aunt tries to tell you about your daughter's lack of table manners. You go into a defensive or resisting mode. Just like the prior story, you need to figure out what you are resisting feeling. Let's say you don't want to feel like a bad mother. Go do your work. Go be quiet and feel what it "feels like" to feel like a bad mother. After you have done the work, your aunt cannot do anything to you that you have not just done to yourself. Who knows? When you go back to your aunt, maybe she has an idea or two that you might really like and you can engage in this conversation without a charge.

Another aspect of "go there" is to anticipate a potential problem that tends to repeat itself in your life, and be prepared for the situation that habitually gives you a charge. You will be amazed at how well this technique works. Let's say your ex-spouse doesn't answer the phone when you call, and you know that he has caller ID. Let's say you need to ask him a question about your child. Have a prior expectation that he will not answer the phone this time, making sure you don't have a charge before you make the call. When you make the call, if he answers, you can be pleasantly surprised. If he doesn't answer, you will not get a charge, because you expected it. Remember, Peace management is aimed at keeping you healthy. The charge means harmful chemicals are circulating in your body.

Changing your expectations does not mean always aiming low, it just means anticipating, in an effort to prevent a charge. Let's take another phone example. Let's say you are behind on several of your bills. You have received repeated phone calls from bill collectors with threatening, provocative words. Every time your phone rings, anticipate it is a bill collector, take a few breaths, maintain your Peace, and then answer the phone. Never allow the bill collector to rob your Peace. It serves no purpose. And who knows, it might even be a call from someone pleasant to talk to instead.

When you use the technique described above or something similar, it is true Peace management. This means that you are protecting your Peace. This is opposed to getting stressed, and needing a stress management technique to pull you back. That's too late. The harmful chemicals have already been released, and the damage is done.

Along this same line, it is always helpful to have a plan B and plan C for anything important. There is a certain psychology to this. If you have the plan B and C in place, you are essentially prepared for things not to go perfectly. Therefore, if you have to resort to another plan, you don't have the emotions associated with failure.

I purposely have a cynic review my material as a way of preparing me for a tough audience. When I get the material back, it is all red and chopped apart. He has critiqued the information like no one else. I appreciate the feedback, so I continue to send it to him. I know what to expect, so I do not get stressed when I see the red ink.

I have implemented Peace management by "going there" ahead of time.

"Going there" means doing the anticipation of a situation in a "safe" manner, before being confronted with the actual situation that in the past, before Peace management, might have given you a charge.

Here are a few examples of "going there" put into use:

- When my best friend and I were on vacation with the kids, her son jumped into the pool, almost on top of her, when she wasn't prepared for it. Her finger nail dug into his head. In a comical yet automatic way, she quickly said "Peace management! I am going to see blood." She is a nurse and quick to react, even in her Peace management! She quickly decided to "go there" to be ready for the eventual reality.

- I have a friend, Rita, who decided to have a conversation with her boss about a decision the boss had made. Rita knew it was going to be a tough conversation, with potential for a great deal of emotion and charge. The bottom line was that Rita felt she had to tell her boss that she could not go ahead with a plan her boss had devised because she felt it was unethical. And no matter how much Rita sugar-coated her comments, she would still be conveying the idea that she felt her boss lacked integrity. Rita called me up and asked how to handle the situation. I told her I did not want to be part of the decision to tell her boss or not tell her boss. That was up to Rita and her gut. However, if she decided to tell her, I would help her with "going there."

  Rita decided to tell her boss. We spent approximately a half hour on the phone, imagining all the possible reactions her boss might have and decided to "go there" by role playing likely scenarios. Of course, we could never anticipate every possible reaction, but we covered enough possible conversations that Rita was ready to maintain her Peace no matter which way her boss reacted.

- My son and I were ready to leave the house for his baseball game. We heard a loud crash upstairs. By the intensity of the sound, we knew something major had happened. I decided to "go there" with my son (in terms of Peace management) before we went to explore physically. I said "that sounded like something major happened. Why don't we go find out what it was, and we will handle it after your game." Sure enough, all the closet racks in my husband's closets had pulled away from the wall. When we saw the mess, there was no charge, no emotion. All we jokingly said was "we hope Gary gets home before us tonight."

- My friend, Steven called. He told me that the technique I call "go there" worked almost too well for him. He and his wife had decided to prepare their son, Travis for his "big boy bed" to prevent any negative emotions. They employed all the elaborate plans many of you probably did in preparing your own children. Well, Travis liked the idea so well that he would not go back to the baby crib. So until the "big boy bed" actually arrived, Steven and his wife took turns camping out on Travis's floor. Steven certainly prevented any stress Travis would experience about losing his crib. Good job Steven! I just hope you have better luck with timing next time!

Here's another example of how anticipating a problem and becoming fully aware of Peace management can serve you well. As you're driving along, suddenly a police cruiser appears behind you. In that instant, you have no idea if he is after you or someone else (or on his way for a donut). Begin to control your breathing with your full attention on the exhalation.

Take care not to take sudden breaths in, as this could tense your muscles and initiate a charge, but truly focus on slow exhalations. This helps you stay relaxed and manage your Peace, preventing a charge. Your body doesn't want to release the harmful chemicals during relaxation. Exhaling helps you relax, so this can actually prevent a charge. Continue the slow exhalations until the officer either passes you or he turns on his red and blue lights. If he pulls you over, try self talk. "Stress is not going to turn back the clock and make me go slower. Stress is not going to get me out of a ticket. Stress will only harm me."

As you will see later, many of my students use visualizations to "go there" and prevent a stress response. You can get very creative in attempting to anticipate situations in an effort to prepare your mind to maintain Peace.

<u>Exercise (S)</u>:

Go There

Goals for this section:

- Whenever you feel yourself defending a position strongly or resisting something, utilize the "go there" technique
- Have an awareness that anticipating and having a plan will truly help you manage your Peace
- Make an actual plan for some of your recurring stressors
- Create an awareness that "going there" during a safe time will prevent the charge in the actual situation

---

<u>Activity A:</u>

This exercise will be used during the heat of the moment. Therefore, just give it some thought now.

Realize there might be times when someone says something to you that provokes a resistant response in you. Be prepared to take an immediate time out. Isolate yourself and truly give time and attention to identifying what you do not want to feel.

Once you identify what you do not want to feel in specific words, actually feel what it is you don't want to feel. Afterwards, say to yourself "that wasn't so bad." Go back to continue the conversation without a charge.

Activity B:

What are some of the recurring situations in your life that cause stress?

For this exercise, you could either "go there" now, allowing yourself to feel what you have resisted feeling

or

at least become cognizant of this concept as you become aware of repeating stressors you encounter.

Determine a very concrete plan for maintaining your Peace in these habitually stressful situations.

Technique: Detachment: Experiencing Life Through Sensory Intake and the Transient Nature of Things

This concept builds on several other techniques and concepts as a way to improve your experiences and minimize your disappointments. It allows you to fully experience all life has to offer, without feeling a need to tightly cling to *things* as your source of joy.

Joy is ever-renewed when you allow yourself to open up and experience whatever life offers you. People often experience fear when they think that they could possibly lose things to which they are attached. They have somehow attached their identity, or more strongly their existence, to things, titles, or labels.

People often attribute their joy or potential joy to something they currently have or plans for what they will have. One way to begin to understand this tendency is to think back to some prior point in your life when things were exciting or fun.

When I was twenty years old, I was newly married, in nursing school, and owned a health club with my husband. I didn't think life could get any better. And if you would have asked me at that time if I ever wanted my life to change, I would have emphatically answered "no." I was attached to the things, labels, and titles I had. Now I look back and appreciate the experience for what it was, but I am also very grateful that my life, circumstances, and labels have changed many times.

When ownership of the complex was changing hands and we were forced to sell the health club, things fell apart. We didn't know the direction our lives would take. It was scary and fear set in. Although I had had prior attachment to the roles, experiences, and titles that I had in high school, I hadn't realized it at the time. Losing the health club was the first time I experienced a loss of something to which I was attached.

If, during the time we owned the health club, I would have realized my "attachment" and focused on the possible loss, I would have experienced anxiety that my life might somehow change. Not only would I have been living life from a place of fear, but I also would not have enjoyed the experiences I was having at the time they were happening. That was exactly what happened in the immediate period following loss of the health club. I became fearful of losing other things.

Luckily, I began to see the detrimental impact of this line of thinking shortly after the health club was sold. Had I not addressed the issue of loss related to attachment, most of my life would have been lived from a place of fear, because my life has been a sequence of doors closing and other ones opening. This also brings up a saying I developed early on that expands on one you probably already know:

When one door closes, another door will open, but don't expect it to look like the door that just closed.

I have usefully applied my thinking about detachment to many areas of my life. At age 26, I was appointed the Assistant Director of Nursing at a local community hospital (and for a few months, at age 27, I was actually in charge of the nursing department while they were searching for another director). My life seemed to change by the minute during that period of time, but I stayed open to all of the experiences. It became an incredible period of growth for me. This wonderful period ended when the hospital brought in outside consultants to help cut costs, as the hospital was in financial jeopardy and losing money. The consultants made changes that I disagreed with on a moral level, so regretfully, I resigned, not having another door waiting for me.

Although I enjoyed my tenure as Assistant Director of Nursing, I was not attached to it. This lack of attachment allowed me to stay centered and calm as I made my decision to leave the hospital and become unemployed. It kept me in the right frame of mind to seek another opportunity.

If I had been attached to my old position, I might have desperately fought to convince the hospital administrators that the nursing consultant was making bad decisions that would cost the hospital more in the long term. I might have stayed there, fighting the fight, which would have been stressful and futile.

On a similar note, often people are attached to their looks. Therefore, they experience much anguish when they gain weight or start to see signs of aging. Except for people who have plastic surgery, there is no way to avoid the signs of aging. You can keep yourself healthy and avoid toxic substances, which will have the benefit of a more youthful appearance, but that is not really the point. The point is the experience of loss because of the attachment to a particular appearance. Those who are not attached to their looks or who are at least accepting of the temporary nature of youth will weather the changes better. Therefore, they will not lose their Peace with the changes.

Although I am aware of the gradual loss of my youth, I am not focused on it. And although I am aware that many people benefit socially from good looks, I am not attached to looks or focused on them. The best example I can share happened several years ago. I was in a bicycle accident. A bad one! I split my face open in two places and had multiple wounds scattered all over my body. Being a teacher, I am in front of groups of students every day.

Believe it or not, because of my detachment from appearance, appearing in public with obvious wounds did not sadden or anger me in the least. However, I am aware of the fact that others are impacted by appearance. When I made it back to class, the first thing I said to my class was "Okay, get it out of the way, spend a minute looking at my face (the asymmetry of my eye brows, the healing gashes and scars), then you will be able to focus on what I am saying and not on the goofy looks." They all chuckled, but we were soon back to teaching and learning.

You set yourself up for failure and loss of Peace when you become attached to anything that is temporary.

Another area that allows us to be robbed of Peace, is to think, "I will have Peace and joy when . . . " (fill in the blank for yourself). Admit it, you probably do this to some extent. It is common for people to blame their lack of happiness during a current time frame on the fact that they haven't made it "there" *yet*, or they haven't acquired some material item *yet*. Have you ever said, "when I get a new job, then I will be happy," or "if I get a new car, then I will be happy," or "when I get pregnant, then I will be happy"?

When you base your happiness on future expectations, you are tying your happiness to an event, person, or thing. All these events or things are transient anyway. Do you really want to tie your happiness to someone or something that will not be around forever? And I am not saying you cannot be happy if you have a new job, or if you have a new car, or if you get pregnant. You can be happy and at Peace with or without them. It is your choice.

I am simply saying that the happiness does not come from the item or event. It comes from the way you decide to experience life. I could be happy and at Peace if I had a vintage Jeep and I am happy and Peace without one now.

You can have fun creating the life you want and acquiring the material things you want, as long as you are not attached to them. The attachment is what brings on the fear and doesn't allow the full experience of a joyful life. This leads to the concept of experiencing life through sensory intake.

Let's go back to the vintage Jeep. I could experience happiness looking at it or feeling the thrill when the top was down and the wind was blowing on me. I could enjoy the smell of fresh cut hay as I was driving around. I would be enjoying the experience through my senses (sight, sound, smell, taste, and touch), not through my mind and what I thought the Jeep would do for me. I wouldn't be enjoying the Jeep when it was in my garage and I was in the office. If I did, that would be an attachment to the Jeep. I would think I was enjoying it with my mind. This could lead to a fear of losing it.

Experiencing through your senses allows you to partake in the temporary joy of a situation, event, or acquisition without holding attachment to it. This is a good thing. It doesn't allow you to erroneously think a thing will give you a permanent sense of joy. Realizing that nothing in the material world is permanent removes the pressure of trying to make it permanent. You can't, and if you really thought about it and were honest with yourself, you probably wouldn't want it to be.

Be open to experiencing all life has to offer without attachment. Don't judge any experience as bad or good. It simply is. Enjoy the fact that everything is transient. This is what allows you to have a full range of experiences in life. Be aware that your sensory intake is what allows you to experience things, and this is what brings you joy.

<u>Exercise (T)</u>:

Detachment: Experiencing Life Through Sensory Intake and the Transient Nature of Things

---

Goals for this section:

- Recognize that everything in the material world is transient or temporary
- Take joy in the transient nature of things
- Identify the things you are hoping for in the future
- Realize the joy you will experience from those desires is attached to the experience, not the acquisitions
- Focus on the sensory experience of life in all circumstances

---

<u>Activity A:</u>

Identify something in the material world that has a guarantee of permanence. Write it down.

Okay, that was a trick. Focus on the empty space above. Realize that there isn't anything in the material world that is guaranteed to be permanent. So let go of trying to make anything permanent.

The only way to experience joy is to realize everything is temporary. So if you want to enjoy life, you have to enjoy it now.

Think of your own life. Realize the stagnation you would feel if things never changed. Embrace change, growth, and the opportunity to experience new things.

Activity B:

List the things you are hoping for in the future (a better job, a new car, a mate)

____

____

____

____

____

Now picture how you will enjoy those additions to your life. Realize, the enjoyment is not from having them, it is from experiencing them.

Imagine how you will experience the additions. This will help you, once you acquire them, to enjoy them in the present and through your senses, as opposed to with your mind.

Activity C:

Take a moment to cultivate an awareness of and make a commitment to allow sensory intake to become the way you experience things. Focus on this throughout the next day.

At the end of the day, ask yourself "did I enjoy life at a higher level this way?".

Technique: *Listen* to your Gut & Listen to your *Gut*

This section pertains to gaining a higher level of awareness of that part of you that has a higher level of intuitive intelligence. Note the emphasis on the different words in the title. In our society, we use the word "gut" to refer to something that guides us at a higher level than our heart or our mind can do alone. When we refer to our gut, we are thinking of a highly refined internal mechanism that knows our every thought, feeling, and desire at a more core level than we can possibly verbalize.

When we learn to tune in to our gut, we have an added dimension to our human system that helps us interpret and make decisions. Everyone has probably had the experience of "listening to their gut" when making a decision. You may even have used these exact words. This technique will allow you to expand on your prior use and help you refine this system.

"*Listen* to your gut" with the emphasis on *listen*, pertains to how we use our gut to interpret information, whereas "listen to your *gut*", with the emphasis on *gut*, pertains to using your gut as part of the decision making process. Let's start with using your gut to help interpret information.

We are constantly bombarded with information, both from external sources (provided by other people and our environment) and from our internal source (the constant stream of thoughts we have that continually add to our mind's data bank). Without even realizing it, we are also continually interpreting this information:

are we accepting this information as valid?
does it become a part of our belief system?
does it become a part of our goals?
does it become a fear?

do we toss it into our internal garbage can?
does it align with our current values, morals and beliefs?

Our gut, or internal interpreting mechanism, addresses these questions automatically. It goes beyond where our "logical" thinking goes and it is not always consistent with ideas that are socially acceptable. In a sense, our gut has a "mind" of its own. Our gut communicates to us if the new information is in line with our core desires. Unfortunately, our gut doesn't speak in words, let alone English. It communicates to us in feelings, but these feelings are relatively subtle.

The feelings of overt Peace-robbing emotions (stress, fear, anger) should be easily recognized by you at this point in the program. You should be easily able to identify your charge. However, we now need to fine tune our emotion-reading mechanism a bit. This technique of *listening* to your gut requires your time and attention. At first, your gut will not be something you can "hear" if you are rushed, in a chaotic situation, or preoccupied. Eventually, you will be so tuned into it, you will always have it on high radar. You will recognize your gut's communication, even if you are in the midst of chaos. In fact, one of the things your gut will probably communicate is "get the heck out of this chaotic situation!"

What is this communication I am referring to? It is basically a black or white, good or bad, yes or no (two answer system) feeling response. Your gut tells you "this is right for you or its wrong for you". Some may call the response of their gut either a "calm" or an "uneasy" feeling.

If you get tuned into this "uneasy feeling" as a type of internal interpretation and communication, you will realize that you need to fix something that is not in balance. You will benefit by learning to interpret your gut, because you cannot analyze your thoughts while you are in the thought. That is impossible. Therefore, if you can increase awareness of the messages sent to you through subtle feelings, you will always know what is good for you. Your gut will tell you when something is wrong. Listen!

Remember, you do not have to see things for them to be real. Can you see temperature? (I am not referring to looking at a thermometer) You cannot see it, but it is there. Therefore, you need more than your eyes to interpret things. You have this extra "sense." Use it. A gut is a terrible thing to waste!

The first phrase, *listen* to your gut implies that the system is always turned "on" (you can't turn it off, although you may choose not to "listen" to it). It is always there for you, should you chose to use this system to serve as a radar for things that are not good for you. However, if you utilize your gut as part of the decision making process, as in the phrase "listen to your *gut*" you consciously call upon this system when you are actively making a decision.

When you are making a decision, you often take advice from others into account, plus you also call upon your past experience, your "heart", and your "mind". This can all be very complex. And you might have also heard the sayings "your heart may steer you wrong" or "your mind can steer you wrong," but I bet you've never heard "your gut will steer you wrong." I believe that is because your gut will *never* steer you wrong. Your gut is very highly refined; it is a form of high level inner intelligence that does not leave out any small details in the decision making process.

The gut is also very highly individualized. Let's say two nurses went on an interview for a job in an intensive care unit. The same nurse manager interviewed both prospective employees. The nurse manager tried to create very stressful interviews, to help her determine if the candidates for the job can handle stress well. I know that if I was in that interview, my gut would be telling me that something was not genuine. I am at a point in my career where I am a little choosy. I might even stop the interview, in a polite way (as I have in the past), because I could tell the job was not a good match for me. My gut would take into account my total situation and tell me not to take the job.

The same situation would possibly be very different for the other nurse. She might be a single mom with three school age children, and this might be the only straight day shift job available. She might have felt the same thing I felt, yet her gut says the tactics of the nurse manager is something she is willing to overlook because her kids need her at home in the evening. Her gut would probably guide her to take the job.

This situation I presented is a very superficial one, in that I only presented a few facts that went into the decision making in this job interview. There will be many more facts, desires, and history that your gut will actually take into consideration. Your gut is very complex and able to take in all the intricacies of your life.

You will eventually get to the point where the process of "following your gut" becomes very natural. You will not actually give it any conscious thought because it becomes the way you make all your big and small decisions. However, at first, the process may be very mechanical. In fact, in the following exercise, I will actually present an exercise you can use when you are learning to tune-into your gut for decision making. Your gut will tell you this decision is good for you or not good for you. There is no gray area for the gut in decision making.

For both interpreting and decision making, you need time, patience, and a willingness to get to know your body and its responses. It will pay off greatly. I can honestly say that when I have made decisions that were from my gut, I have never looked back and said "boy, I shouldn't have done that." But there have been plenty of times when my gut said one thing, but I did something else and paid dearly. I have a feeling you can relate to this.

<u>Exercise (U)</u>:

Listen to your Gut

Goals for this section:

- Increase awareness of the subtle messages of your gut as you carry on day-to-day activities
- Utilize information from your gut in your decision making process

---

<u>Activity A:</u>

For the next day, make a conscious effort to be highly aware of your feelings, especially the subtle ones. Try to stop yourself periodically to do a "feeling check." Do you feel an easiness or an uneasiness?

Notice if you are catching yourself in a feeling state, without the need to do these periodic "feeling checks." The more you turn your awareness to your gut, the quicker it will be utilized as your radar.

Determine if you feel in balance with life or out of balance. Whenever you feel an uneasiness, STOP. Learn to recognize that uneasiness is a message from your gut that you should heed. It is a form of training. Take it slowly, but don't allow uneasiness to go unattended.

Activity B:

Practice using your gut to make all of your decisions. If this is a new concept for you, try the following exercise:

You must be alone and in quiet when you are beginning to learn to tune into your gut for decision making. Take any issue you are currently trying to decide. You will make statements, then wait and watch the body response.

You may want to practice with some easy questions (where you actually know what is good for you) first, to understand how your body responds to things that are good for you and bad for you.

Let's say you are considering ending a relationship. Let's say you have been dating a kind man, but there are differences between the two of you that keep creating conflict. You love him, but are finding the situation difficult.

Start with an easy statement. Say "Tim is a kind man." Watch what happens in your body. Probably a relaxing, a settling in your body, or a feeling of expanding.

Then say, "I love Tim." Probably the same response.

Now the hard ones. Say "I should give Tim another chance to work this out." If you feel the same response, your gut is telling you it is the right decision. If you feel a tightening, constricting, or contracting feeling, your gut is probably telling you that you should not give the relationship another chance.

Next, try the statement worded differently (they need to be statements, not questions). Say "It would be best if I end the relationship." If you feel a relaxation, you know your gut "thinks" you should end it.

What is your reaction to using this technique? Are you willing to perfect this technique? If so, use it often in the beginning. You will get to the point where you don't even have to make the statements. You will automatically know the answers from a deep level.

Technique: Is It Really Second Best?

This technique acknowledges the fact that there is often a discrepancy between the way things are, and the way things would be if we could create our ideal world. This creates a great deal of vague stress for us. I say "vague" because it is not related to a single identifiable event. It is more in relation to the general feel of our life.

Above, I used the phrase, "*if* we could create our ideal world". That is a little misleading, because on one level, we *do* create our ideal world—and it is in our *mind* that we create it. Let's go to an example:

> In our ideal world, there is an intact family, one where the biological mother and father have a loving relationship and live in the same house with their two kids. The mom drives a mini van. The father has a very successful job. The husband takes his wife out to dinner every Saturday night. They talk about plans for the future and an enjoyable retirement together.

We play that picture over and over in our mind. It becomes the benchmark for evaluating the quality of our reality. Now, let's say there was a divorce, or the inability to conceive, necessitating adoption. Life doesn't look exactly like our ideal world. We may not give it this exact thought or label, but it is that vague discrepancy between our reality and our ideal world that causes us stress and robs our Peace.

The story of Catherine, a former neighbor, illustrates this exact scenario. She is very family-oriented by nature and desire. She definitely values that "Leave it to Beaver," all-American family. However, she is divorced. Therefore, that perfect family that she desires is no longer an option. Catherine has two wonderful, healthy children. She owns a thriving antique store. And her current husband is a gem by all measurements. Unfortunately, this is her fourth husband and she is only 38 years old. She has been chasing the dream that can no longer be fulfilled, simply because of the fact that the biological father and mother of her children cannot live in the same home. She has tried desperately to create that ideal. But any family she has will never measure up exactly to what she believes is ideal.

Another friend, Barb, had several miscarriages, two of which were ectopic pregnancies, where the babies grew inside her tubes instead of the uterus. Both of these required removal of the tubes. She had to adopt children if she wanted to be a mother. Barb has two beautiful children from Russia. These children are bright and loving, and one is even gifted in music. Barb often expresses to me the guilt she feels for having thoughts of wishing they were her biological children.

I can relate to feeling a discrepancy. I also value an intact family and realize the optimal situation would have been for my ex-husband and I to stay married and raise our son under one roof. That simply did not happen. I experienced that stress from the discrepancy between my reality and my ideal.

The strategy that helped me and is helping the women described above is called "is it really second best?". My hope is that Catherine can work through this one quickly, before she releases another husband because of something he is unable to provide for her: her ideal world.

The first step is simply acknowledging the discrepancy and labeling it for what it is. It requires some work, but the Peace it brings is well worth it! You must spend time analyzing the picture that you call or feel is "perfect."

The next step is looking at your current situation and all the blessings you have in that situation. It is the situation that you are currently living and experiencing. You must acknowledge the discrepancy between your life and your ideal (including all the blessings) and realize in that particular comparison, it *is* second best. But in reality, it is probably *the best* it could be for the time. I am not suggesting that you would even call your life wonderful or good right now. It might be or it might not be. It is just the best given your circumstances.

I do not suggest giving up thoughts of your ideal. You actually did a great deal of work throughout your life creating that perfect picture. It is a culmination of all your heart's desires played out in one "movie clip." It is the sum total of all your intentions, wishes, or desires. That picture is very valuable to you, giving your life direction and focus. It provides the map for how you will make decisions in your life, in an attempt to move closer to that ideal picture.

The harm that comes from playing that picture is the *stress* that is felt when you focus on the discrepancy, rather than moving your life so that it is more closely aligned with your picture. In using the picture to assist with creating the life that you want, first acknowledge any areas that can no longer be, simply by virtue of your circumstances.

In my case, I am a divorced mother. I will never be able to provide a home for my son where his biological parents live in the same house and share life experiences. All three of us living together would be part of my ideal. However, I have a healthy son, who keeps me challenged and focused on enjoying life. I have a loving husband. He is a loving and responsible step-father who values family time. He has a stable job. He is a man of his word and brings fun and joy to my life. I have a job where I feel I make a difference and contribute to my profession. I have friends who share enjoyment of activities with me and provide a network of caring and emotional support. My "second best" which in reality, *is* my best, is pretty darn good.

Once you have established gratitude for your current life, you can identify ways in which you can more closely align your current life with your ideal. I no longer waste my time or experience negative emotions grieving the inability to have my perfect picture. Rather, I experience gratitude and joy for the life I am living. This brings me Peace, and that is my real goal!

Some of you may be ready to pull out your hair at this point, thinking that I didn't acknowledge how far away from ideal you currently are. I was there too! In this case, you are actively working toward that "best in reality." It can happen for you! But you must remain at Peace while you work toward your best reality.

For those of you who feel a wide disparity between your ideal and your current life, just realize you are in a process that can be used to move you closer to that ideal through carefully making choices in your life.

For those of you who are not that far off from your "ideal," this technique was meant for you. There are two ways in which you could be slightly off your ideal. First, you might have your perfect life on paper, but lack the feeling of connection with one or more of your family members. Or a few of the circumstances of your life (e.g. never married, adopted children, single parent, an alcoholic spouse) are not part of your ideal picture. If you move through this process, making choices that lead you closer to your ideal when possible, you will replace that vague feeling of stress with a new found Peace about your current life.

Spend some time in the following exercise getting a handle on the discrepancy, moving toward gratitude, and making decisions that will move you closer to your ideal. This is what will aid in bringing you Peace.

Exercise (V):

Is it Really Second Best?

Goals for this section:

- Acknowledge at some level you have a "perfect picture" of your life that lives in your mind
- Get in touch with the specific details of that ideal picture
- Give thought to your real life and identify all the areas of discrepancy between your ideal and real life
- List all the wonderful things in your life, the areas for which you feel gratitude
- Identify areas in your life which are under your control and that you are able to change
- Think of decisions you may make in your future that can bring you closer to your ideal picture
- Experience gratitude for your current life and for the fact that you have the ability to work toward your ideal situation if you choose

---

Activity A:

You need about 15 minutes of undisturbed quiet time to answer the questions in this exercise.

1. Do you have some idea or concept of what your ideal life would look and feel like?

2. What are the circumstances and who are the players of that life?

In analyzing that *ideal life*, here some questions you may ask yourself:

- does your marital status matter?
- if so, are you married or single?
- are there children in your life?
- if so, do the children need to be biologically yours? (remember, in your ideal situation)
- what are your relationships like with these family members?
- what kind of activities do you do alone and with these people?
- what kind of job do you have, or are you retired?
- if you work, how do you feel about that job?
- how many close friends do you have?
- what are those relationships like?
- how is your relationship with your extended family?
- what is your financial situation?
- how much money do you have in the bank?
- what is your financial plan for your retirement?
- where do you live?
- what kind of a house do you live in?
- what kind of car do you drive?
- what do you do to nourish yourself emotionally, physically, and/or spiritually?

Add in anything else that completes your picture.

Activity B:

Now ask yourself the same questions about your *real life*. As you go along, make a mental note of all the discrepancies.

Activity C:

Even though you probably already acknowledge that your life is not perfect or close to your ideal, list the things in your real life for which you experience genuine gratitude.

Activity D:

Use a pencil for this exercise.

Go back to your two descriptions, that of your ideal world and that of your real world. What are the actual discrepancies? List them below. Then identify which items are important and which items are not important. Once you list which items are important, determine why they are important. If during this process you find they are really not important, put the check mark in the "not important" column.

Discrepancy	important	not important

Activity E:

Recopy the list of the above discrepancies that are important to you. Determine if you are able to change them or not.

Important Discrepancies	Able to Change or Not

Activity F:

Given the list above (from activity E) write a possible plan for achieving those desired changes that are within your ability to change.

Activity G:

Spend a moment in gratitude for

- your current life
- having the knowledge of the discrepancies
- knowledge of which areas are in your ability to change
- for having the time to give conscious thought to choosing the direction of your life.

Become aware of the Peace and power you feel for having had these revelations and growth opportunity.

Technique: Visualizations

This technique will allow a great deal of your own creativity. I do not personally use visualizations but many of my students do and they often share their use of visualization in practicing Peace. Therefore I created group exercises for my students. Included are a few examples as a way to start you on your own path, if this is something that works for you.

- One student recently went through a divorce. Whenever her ex-husband came to pick up the children, he would say things that most of us would interpret as very cruel. Donna said that it felt as though his words were like daggers cutting into her. The visualization she now uses when her ex-husband speaks is that she sees his words as feathers floating out of his mouth. The feathers always float to the floor before they can get to her. She says she experiences an inner smile and feels Peace as she gains control of her emotion and images.

- Another student told the class she had extreme difficulty and stress when dealing with her mother-in-law. Her mother-in-law picks up her children after school, and Maria needed to go over to her mother-in-law's house three times a week to pick up her children. She needed a technique to manage her Peace. She said that as soon as she would pull onto her mother-in-law's street, she would visualize placing a "Peace shield" around herself. Then, when she would enter her mother-in-law's home, she would visualize that nothing her mother-in-law would say could penetrate her shield. No matter how harsh or critical her mother-in-law was, Maria was able to maintain her Peace.

- Finally, one student who had severe test anxiety utilized visualization. This was a bright young woman, who was a sharp, clear thinker in the hospital setting. But when a written test was put in front of her, she froze. She said the test controlled her.

Her strategy was that while driving to school on the morning of a test, she imagined her car was a steam roller for Peace. She was able to roll over anything that blocked her from being successful. She said that by the time she got to school, she felt so confident, that she excitedly waited for her test to be handed to her. As a result, she was more successful once she started using this technique than she had been in any previous courses.

Although I do not utilize this technique, you can see the effectiveness it can have. I encourage you to create your own visualizations, as many have found them very helpful.

Exercise (W):

Visualization

Goals for this section:

- Identify areas of your life where visualization could help you manage your Peace
- Create visual images you can call upon as a strategy for managing your Peace

---

Activity A:

Identify areas in your life which seem repeatedly to bring you opportunities to practice Peace.

Activity B:

Take those trouble areas and visualize either an image or a mini movie clip that you can play in your mind the next time you encounter that troubling situation.

Technique: Deal With It or Let it Go

"Deal with it or let it go." These are the words that just came out of my mouth as I spoke to one of my nursing students. We'll call her Sara. Sara is a sharp cookie, but she is currently less than successful in my course. It is a tough, rigorous, time-consuming course, but I have had students who have not been as talented as Sara pass my course successfully.

Sara is on the tail end of her divorce proceeding. She is raising three small children, and she just failed one of her other courses. She has many plates spinning, but I still sensed there was something I was missing. I knew that despite what was going on in Sara's life, she could be successful in my class.

Indeed there was. Sara is truly devastated by failing another class. The failure has put her behind schedule for graduation, which will not allow her to make the necessary money to keep her head above water. In fact, she may lose her house. She has thought about filing a grievance at the college to get some decisions reversed, but she hasn't done so. I don't know the specifics, but she feels there was some wrong-doing. I had the feeling that filing a grievance was not really her intention, but that she was being pulled down by having that option.

Actually, being distracted by life decisions plagued Sara during the course that she failed. There were other decisions about her life that needed to be made during that course. The decisions preoccupied her mind so much, that she ended up not giving the required time and attention to that course. Now she is in my course, but only physically. I say that because her mind is still in the other course that she failed. She is not "present" and engaged in the moment at hand. To say Sara is preoccupied with failing her last course is putting it mildly. She is now more light hearted about the matter than in the first week of my course, now often joking about it.

Yet, the issue still occupies most of her conversations and interactions with others.

I finally pulled Sara aside and told her she needed to make a choice. And believe it or not, I was not asking her to choose Peace. She was not ready for this yet. I asked her to "deal with it or let it go," meaning file the grievance or let it go. Thinking about it without action was only dragging her down. The issue was all-consuming. Sara either needed to pursue the action of a grievance or *not give it another thought*. Her focus on the decision about not having filed a grievance and failing the course took her attention off the present and put her attention on the past, *where events are not changeable*! During our conversations, Sara kept trying the "yeah, but" approach. I won't go to the, "yeah, but" and didn't let Sara go there either. That would serve no purpose in this type of situation. It is very clear that Sara needs to make a choice to deal with the situation or let it go. If she doesn't make a choice, she will stay in limbo and will be tormented continuously. This is truly an example of robbing Peace.

I would like to share a story I found in a magazine years ago, and kept for many years on my refrigerator door. I still have it in my Daytimer and keep it close at hand. The tale goes like this:

> Two monks were traveling along and came to a stream with a beautiful maiden beside it trying to get across. One of the monks lifted the maiden onto his back, carried her across, and set her down on the other side. She thanked him and the monks continued along their way. After a while, one monk turned to the other.
>
> "Didn't you break your vows of chastity and celibacy by carrying that beautiful maiden?" he asked his companion.
>
> The other monk replied, "Oh, are you still carrying her? I set her down a long time ago."
>
> The message was unambiguous: Get out of the past. Don't wallow in old feelings. Each

moment is fresh. Do what needs to be done today.
Pay attention to the now.

I loved this story twenty years ago, and it is still valuable to me today. I often share this story with people who are hanging on to the past, at the cost of missing the present. There is no time more precious than the present, and it is the only time in which you can experience the bliss of Peace. You cannot *experience* Peace in the past. You cannot *experience* Peace in the future. You can only experience the magnificence of Peace in the present. If you allow yourself to be plagued by the past or immobilized with fear of the future, you are robbed of enjoying Peace in the present.

This thief of Peace (not choosing to either deal with something or let it go) is different than suffering. This does not necessarily represent an emotional burden, but it does invade your time and energy, preventing a still mind. This, like suffering, requires analyzing any lack of Peace. Determine if there are any situations which need to be brought to a decision.

Exercise (X):

Deal With it or Let it Go

Goals for this section:

- Identify any areas that consume your time and attention, including pending decisions, not allowing you to experience Peace
- Make a conscious decision to deal with something that is bothering you, either by taking action or letting the matter go

---

Activity:

Whenever you are in a moment that feels like the absence of Peace,

A) examine if your mind is focusing on things from the past that

- can be addressed through some form of action to alter the course of the future

- cannot be changed by any form of action

If you identified something that can be addressed through some form of action, and you choose to deal with it,
begin that action now,

if not, then **let it go**

If you identified something that cannot be changed by any course of action

let it go

B) examine if your mind is focusing on something that may occur in the future

- Can action alter the course to assure a favorable result?

- Is there *no action* that can assure a favorable result?

If an action can alter the course of events favorably, begin that action now,

if not, - **let it go**

Technique: Take Charge of the Sadness

The topic of sadness caused the biggest delay in the progress of this book. It is easy to identify sadness as a negative emotion, because it is not a positive one; sadness makes you feel bad, not good. I was stuck on this topic because, initially, I felt Peace management was a program of strategies aimed at ridding people from all negative emotions. Yet something inside me was saying, "sadness is not an emotion we want to abolish from our existence."

I researched sadness, both in literature and the anecdotal experiences of those in my circle. Then in a quiet moment, it came to me. There is no need to try to manage your Peace in a way that doesn't allow the emotion of sadness to enter. Sadness is what keeps us in touch with our humanness. We need to honor this emotion.

A good Peace manager allows sadness to be experienced in a healthy way. Sadness is often equated with the feeling of grieving. Grieving is what we experience as a reaction to loss. Most of the time we associate the loss with death, but it could be in relation to any loss, (e.g. loss of health, loss of a spouse through divorce, loss of a job, loss of family unity). I feel that if we did not allow ourselves to feel sadness, we would not be authentic in our emotions.

There is a kind of immobilizing sadness, though, that I could not support. You are probably aware of this type of sadness. It is the kind that seems insidiously to creep into your every waking moment. The following visualization may help you identify the unhealthy sadness that we will want to take charge of and contain:

> For some, sadness is like an invisible weed or vine that attaches itself to the body and wraps itself around and around, entangling and ensnaring the person. As it continues to grow on itself, it seems as though it eventually penetrates the skin and infiltrates

> the inner body. Once inside, it seems to wrap itself around vital organs. Eventually it seems to strangle and suffocate any last, remaining feelings of happiness or Peace.

Obviously, this would be unhealthy. Well, what do you do about it? (This is probably a good time to mention that if this sadness is not simply a sadness, but possibly a clinical depression, it would be best to seek professional attention to determine need for therapy or medications). But once it is determined to be sadness, you must first acknowledge it for what it is. You acknowledge that sadness has taken on a life of its own and unfortunately, it is your life that it has taken on (and taken over).

The second step is to take charge of the sadness, putting yourself in the drivers seat, in terms of how and when you experience it. One simple technique has worked well for me and most everyone I counsel in this area. I call it "isolating the sadness."

Let's say you are washing dishes and actually enjoying the moment. Then out of the blue, you are consumed with the sadness related to the break-up of a relationship. You need to realize that sadness has taken over, then begin the process of isolation. Begin by identifying someplace at home (and probably someplace at work, if this sadness interferes with your attention at work), where you can isolate yourself from activity. For me, it is a glider outside my home office.

Once you identify that sadness has taken over, you need to go sit in that place, and really be with the sadness while you are there. You need to feel it and try to identify what specifically has created the sadness. You need to stay in your place until you have worked through the sadness for this moment. When you feel better, go back to washing the dishes. Enjoy the view out your window, or the breeze coming through the screened window. Continue with your activities. As soon as the feeling of sadness resurfaces, begin the isolation again.

I have a cousin who very painfully lost her best friend in a traumatic accident. Once the shock and anger subsided, I taught her this technique. She said that she spent about 75% of the first weekend in her chair. And the next week, she said her co-workers probably thought she had major gastrointestinal problems. She would isolate herself in the bathroom because it was the only quiet place in her work setting.

My cousin shared her progress with me. She said that she spent about 50% of her time in the chair during the following weekend. She said that her time in the chair gradually decreased over time, until most of her time was spent at Peace. She admited to occasionally needing the chair, usually late in the evening. She said that very early in this isolation process, she lost the feeling that the sadness had immobilized her. This happened once she knew that she was in charge of her sadness and able to isolate it. I also believe the sadness is dealt with more effectively when you isolate it, because you force yourself to really look at the issues closer and sooner. You actually are with the sadness more, feeling it more, and working through it more efficiently.

Isolating yourself in a chair 50 -75% of the time may seem like a waste of time. But if you don't do this during a period of immobilizing sadness, it will encompass *more than* 50 - 75% of your life and you will not experience any Peace-full time. However, your situation may not permit you to sit in isolation for a prolonged period of time. I still advocate isolating the sadness, but you may have to be creative in your approach.

I asked my students to come up with a plan if sadness crept in while they were reading or studying for a test. One group of students suggested leaving the book for the time being. They noted that if they were distracted by anything, sadness included, they would keep reading the same material over and over and not a bit of it would sink in. However, they also all agreed that they can not afford to sit in a chair for even 5 minutes if it is a night before an exam.

My students suggested switching activities if sadness crept in while they were studying. They felt they could use that time to do mindless tasks. They allowed themselves to feel sadness during these tasks only. They said they could pack the lunches for the next day or fold laundry. But when they were done with that task they would have to leave the sadness alone for a bit. They realize isolating sadness while performing the mindless tasks is not optimal, but it is very functional given their time constraints. They can then return to their studies with a clear, unrestrained mind. Many students have tried this technique and given high kudos to the group of students who formulated the idea.

I shared the concept of isolating the sadness with a 44 year old woman who was dying of lung cancer. She shared something with me that was equally as valuable. She was told that she had "between 6 months to two years to live." She has a 16 year old son and a 14 year old daughter. Her husband was also dealing with his own chronic illness. The woman shared an incredible technique with me. She would leave the computer on in her home office 24 hours a day. When she became sad or introspective, she would journal on the computer. Her children would also journal or interact with their mother on the computer. They would write their feelings, reflect on what their mother had written, ask her questions, and express their anger in ways they could not share while looking directly into their mother's eyes. Sometimes, they would note that their writings were in the early hours of the morning when they couldn't fall back to sleep.

The members of this family were isolating their sadness to their time on the computer. The rest of their time, they enjoyed the present moment together. I thanked the woman for sharing this lovely idea with me and assured her that her idea would probably be a gift to other families dealing with similar issues.

There is an internal power you will feel as you master self control. Taking charge of your sadness, not allowing it to creep into your every waking moment, will keep sadness in the place it needs to be. Appreciate your sadness. It is the price we pay for loving and living.

Before I leave the topic of sadness, I would like to share a story with you that a mother read to me during her period of grief. She wasn't sure of the source, as it was given to her anonymously:

> There was a parade of happy little children, marching through heaven with lighted candles. Off to the side was one sad little child. The children from the parade called for the sad little child to join them. The child answered "I can't. Every time I try to light my candle, my mother puts it out with her tears."

The following exercise will only need to be utilized during periods of overwhelming sadness. Therefore, I suggest just reading through the exercise if you do not need it at this time, in hopes that you will remember the technique should the need arise.

Exercise (Y):

Take Charge of the Sadness

Goals for this section:

- Identify when your Peace is being robbed because of overwhelming thoughts associated with sadness
- Utilize the isolation techniques during periods of sadness
- Make a mental note of the gradual decline in amount of time spent with sad thoughts
- Evaluate your progress dealing with overwhelming sadness

Activity A:

Make a list of all of the things that currently cause you sadness and rob your Peace.

____

____

____

____

____

____

Activity B:

How often does sadness creep into your life?

Do you feel you are in control of the sadness, or do you feel the sadness is in control of you?

When sadness creeps in, utilize the isolation technique. Make a note of how much time you are spending in isolation. Track the amount of time you are spending in isolation. Do you see the amount of time decreasing? Is the intensity decreasing?

Do you find that isolating the sadness helps to put you in control of how and when the sadness is experienced? Do you notice if you are having more time for joy and Peace as you progress through the process?

A gentle reminder: if you feel, or someone close to you suggests that you may be experiencing clinical depression, please seek out professional assistance.

Technique: Release the Past because of Gratitude

Because of my focus on the Moment or the Now, I am often questioned on the topic of learning from the past. I do agree that we learn from the past and that it is valuable. I also am very thankful for my past, because it has created the current me.

After one session with my students in which we discussed "Peace from the Moment," (the next technique presented in the book), one student asked me "Are we going to talk about how to apply this to our childhood troubles?" I simply said "No." I think this surprised her. I did eventually follow with an explanation.

You cannot create Peace in the past. That is impossible. You can only learn from it, in an attempt to move toward Peace in the Now. And this does not mean dwelling on it, over and over and over. This is a mistake that most of us make. I feel we can learn from the past simply because we experienced it. We incorporate all our past lessons into the "current me," without really needing to give the experiences or lessons a lot of conscious thought. The current me reflects the fact that I have taken something from my past. Giving the past more thought doesn't usually bring about more or better revelations. Thinking about it over and over again is not going to make me learn more. I am done with that lesson.

I have a friend who had a brief marriage that brought her a great deal of pain and sorrow. Karen seems to give a great deal of time and attention to her marriage, divorce, and the lessons she learned from it. However, what I sense in her, is that she has a belief that if she *keeps* giving her past time and attention, she will understand it better. She carries a fear that she will make the same kind of bad choice in the future. I sincerely believe she has already learned all she will learn from that lesson. She has already given "her mistake" a *great deal* of insightful thought. I can almost guarantee she will not make the same mistake again. I wish she could see that all of this additional thought is not making her a better decision maker. She is not acquiring any new revelations. It is simply robbing her Peace.

The best way to learn is through experience. I am sure your parents gave you many warnings to shield you from life's harshest lessons. Did you learn from their words, or did you learn the lesson when you went through situations on your own? I know the answer. In fact, that is the attitude I have in raising my son. I do not try to protect him from life lessons. Rather, I teach him how to be a good decision maker and give him whatever support he needs as he progresses through stages of life lessons.

I have had what some may call, terrible things, in my past, things that no one would ever feel like they could or would want to deal with. It simply was my past. I am the current me largely because of those life experiences and lessons. Period. I am actually grateful for my past, because it has lead to the current me. I like the current me even better than the one I was 5 or 10 years ago. This feeling of success prevails, in large part, because of my willingness to release the past.

I realize that destructive patterns may have developed over the course of your life, and some of you have experienced horrific traumas. I simply ask, does dwelling on the past resolve the dysfunctional patterns or reverse the trauma?

While we are going through something uncomfortable, it is hard to realize that it is a situation that might create a better me in the future. It would be great to realize it while it was happening, but that is a difficult skill to incorporate. It is one I am currently working on myself. I will be a different me 10 years from now, because of what I am going through right now, and because of all the associated life lessons. One of the professors where I teach had a poster outside her door. It said "Oh no, not another life lesson." I chuckled, because my first response was probably the same as yours. However, as I step back, I am actually grateful for all experiences. There is no other way to create yourself than through experience and the resulting growth. Another related quote I heard once was "a transition doesn't feel like a transition, it feels like a crisis."

Some psychologists practice under the philosophy of the need to analyze the past in order to help the present and future. They spend much time analyzing the past. I am not trained in psychology, I am only coming from my gut and my experience working with people in Peace management. If I were a psychologist, I would have to research and utilize a framework that would allow me to gather basic information about my patients' past, for the purpose of understanding them better as people. But that would be the extent of it. I would not do any "work" with the past. I am sure I may get psychologists who will try to argue with me. They can criticize this technique all they want. I simply am not going there. Different people have different philosophies. Period. I just simply don't buy into that philosophy. It doesn't work for me or for the people I counsel in Peace management.

I realize psychiatrists deal with other, very specific patient populations. I could not begin to understand their modalities. But I would find it very rewarding if they could utilize Peace management in addition to the medications they prescribe and other modalities they use.

One very dramatic experience I had with one of my former students was unfortunately prior to my development of Peace management. However, it illustrates how strongly I feel about the lack of benefit from dwelling on, analyzing, and in this case, "re-living" the past. I will call this student Sue. Sue was already a registered nurse who was attending my class as part of her work toward a Bachelor's Degree. She was a very successful nurse manager in a very busy unit. Unfortunately, immediately prior to starting my class, she had been diagnosed with multiple personalities. I admit, this disorder is far beyond my expertise. In fact, while Sue was in my class, I read everything I could get my hands on related to multiple personalities. This was a very unstable period for Sue, as this was a new diagnosis.

With Sue's permission, I had a few limited conversations with her psychiatrist, because of the possible interference his plan would create for Sue's progress in school at this point. We all agreed that Sue would continue with school, but we would evaluate the plan periodically. I in no way felt in a position to challenge what I thought was a very aggressive plan for Sue. Therefore, I simply created the school plan and supported her therapy plan the best I could. However, from the depths of my soul, I felt the treatment plan was too aggressive and questioned its benefit.

Sue confided in me that her past was horrible. Her family was part of a Satanic cult. Her grandfather was the High Priest of the cult and as a teenager, she was what she called "a breeder." I can't even begin to go into the moral implications and horrific details. What does matter, though, is the plan Sue's psychiatrist laid out for her. He had her return to Pennsylvania, to the site where this all occurred, and do some emotional homework.

After that visit there was a terrible change in Sue. She could no longer focus, cope, or do simple daily functions—let alone function as a mother, nurse manager, and student. She was hospitalized twice during the semester, once, for something called body memories. It was explained to me that Sue took on the actual physical pain from her teenage years.

My goal was not to challenge the psychiatrists' comprehensive treatment plan for Sue. Plus, I am certain that I did not have all the facts to have a true understanding of his intentions. But I do know that I came away having a deep regret that I had a part in Sue's trip to Pennsylvania by allowing her to miss a class to participate in this "psychiatric homework." I think this reliving of the past was very detrimental to the emotional health of Sue.

I have lost touch with Sue. I have no way of knowing if the psychiatrist's plan of analyzing and working through the past has had any long term benefit for her. I realize that the fact that she had multiple personalities complicates this case. Sue's is an extreme case. But I hope I was able to use this to illustrate that the analysis of the past came nowhere close to giving Sue Peace in the Moment.

To have Peace in the Moment, we must release the past. To promote the release, you should begin with gratitude for the "current me." Remember, I am the current me because of all of my past experiences. You must acknowledge any past events that are weighing you down in the Now.

Once you identify something that is weighing you down and robbing your Peace, you will need to "be with it" for a while. A former office mate had great difficulty getting pregnant. She underwent many years of testing, treatments, and surgeries. She experienced great anguish. Today, through the technology of in vitro fertilization, she has lovely, six year old twins. She admits that she still "feels a pit in her stomach" when she thinks about all her infertility issues. This is a charge. She is an incredible mother. I can't help but think that, in part, she is such a great mom because of her difficulty in conceiving. She truly values her children and sees her maternal role as a gift. My hope is that she will get to a point where thoughts of the past infertility hold no pain for her, because they have helped her in her current role as a mom.

You can also proceed in reverse, making you more conscious of the concept of gratitude. Currently, I have a decent level of financial savvy. I am very thankful for my knowledge and comfort in this area. This was not always the case. In fact, one conversation I had with my father when I had just separated from my ex husband is laughable now. I asked my father, "how will I know when to pay the bills?" Now, looking back, I am sure he wanted to put his head down, cover his eyes, and shake his head. But he very kindly said, "don't worry, honey. They will just come in the mail."

In my first marriage, I didn't do any of the finances or investing. I simply wrote out a check for the grocery store, not even doing the subtraction after I wrote out the check. During my separation, I was lost! I had no concept of budgeting or saving, let alone investing. Well, I took charge. I took every personal finance course offered locally. I bought several books and magazine subscriptions, and went to lectures. I talked to several financial advisors and analysts. Plus, I became empowered to take charge of my finances by modeling myself after a gentleman I was dating. He had a master's degree in finance and was a CFO. He was very in charge of his finances and his financial future.

Like I said, today I have a good sense of finances. In fact, one of my financial advisors left his job of 20 years to move to a company I told him about. He is having a great deal of career success now. I also started a financial education and support group for women. All of this because of my past: my lack of knowledge, being thrust into a situation where I felt ignorant and powerless, and then the subsequent education. I am thankful for the current me, because of my past lessons.

As you read about releasing the past because of gratitude, did you give it any other label? I did, but I did not want to introduce it before I explained the concept. I did not want any former blocks that you may have associated with this label or word, to continue to block you now. Does this feel anything like "forgiveness"? Many of us have grown up knowing forgiveness was the key to happiness or Peace. This notion might have been conveyed through your religion, your parents, or teachers. It is something I heard many times through out my life, yet it was something that did not resonate with me.

I use to feel that if I forgave someone it meant that either

- I had to "forget" what the other person did to me and therefore was communicating that I did not think the other person wronged me,

or

- I felt it put me in a one-up position. I felt as though I should say, "I forgive you" with my nose in the air, in a way. This did not work for me!

Forgiveness, as it is presented in "Releasing the Past because of Gratitude", does not create either of the above feelings for me. It is forgiving or releasing from a good place. And the benefit is Peace. And without forgiveness you cannot have Peace.

I challenge you to spend some time with the next exercise, coming to a place of gratitude for the current you, then letting go of the past. You are the current you because of it. Work toward letting go and experiencing a sense of appreciation for your life lessons.

Exercise (Z):

Release the Past because of Gratitude

Goals for this section:

- Identify areas from your past which rob your Peace
- Analyze ways you have grown into the current you because of those life experiences
- Feel gratitude for the growth you have had (creation of the current you)
- Release thoughts of the past and any related negative emotions

---

Activity A:

Make a list of all of the things from your past which rob your Peace. (They could be from your childhood or recent past):

1. ______________________________

2. ______________________________

3. ______________________________

4. ______________________________

5. ______________________________

6. ______________________________

If you are like most, you may need an additional sheet of paper.

Activity B:

Take each item above and write down an acknowledgment about the current you—who are you today because of the way you have grown due to that life lesson.

1. ______________________________

____

____

2. ______________________________

____

____

3. ______________________________

____

____

4. ______________________________

____

____

5. ______________________________

____

____

6. ____

____

____

Activity C:

Take a moment to experience genuine gratitude for the growth you have had. Acknowledge its relationship to your past.

Activity D:

Release any negative emotions you carry about the past in relation to each above item. Make a commitment to yourself to permanently change the way you view your past in relation to each item.

Activity E:

Many have found this next exercise a fun and enlightening journey. Do it either as a mental exercise or get the pencil to the paper or the fingers on the computer.

It is time to tell the story of your life. It needs to be titled like this:

"The happy ending story of (insert your name)".

This allows the focus to be on how the events of your life lead to a happy ending. As silly as this exercise sounds, it is very worthwhile in analyzing how your past lead to the current you. Think of some of the great biographies and autobiographies you have read. They are often full of struggles, crisis, and overcoming difficulties.

The last page will bring you up to the current you. The last sentence will read “and s/he lived happily ever after, but that didn’t mean there were no more obstacles or hurdles. It did mean that there was tremendous growth, joy and Peace.

Technique: Peace in the "Moment"

Some call this concept the "Now," some call it the "Present", but I prefer to call it the "Moment" because of the origin of my thinking in relation to this concept. However, I will use these terms interchangeably. I sought this type of Peace long before people came into my path who so eloquently describe this concept. Therefore, I needed to explore it on my own and give it a name that had meaning to me.

What I have since found is that there is a great deal of writing about "being in the Moment" under the various names given to the concept. I have utilized my own philosophies and piggybacked onto other writers' philosophies, in creating a framework for managing Peace.

"In the Moment" is where we experience Peace. There are essentially two things that allow us to be pulled out of "the Moment." They are

(1) *negative emotions* with their associated thoughts

(2) *missing* the Moment, because of a continual focus on or "living" in the past or future. First, we will focus on missing "the Moment."

Years ago, I dated a lovely man, Craig, who brought many gifts of insight into my life. I am extremely grateful that our lives touched. Yet there was one aspect of his persona that created a negative energy. I allowed myself to absorb this energy and by doing so, gave away my Peace.

Craig was brilliant, a financial and mathematical genius. He was always thinking about numbers, finances, and new projects. This was very interesting and intriguing at first. But very soon, I began to realize that this preoccupation was actually a part of something bigger that was creating a vague, unsettled feeling for me.

Finally, one day while Craig was deep in thought as he was working on some financial papers, the wind slammed the door shut. He had a very exaggerated, startled response. It struck me as a little unusual, but I did not say a word about it at that time. Later that day, a few ideas came to me. Once I was able to put my ideas into words, I discussed them with Craig.

Outwardly, Craig appeared to be a very calm man, yet I sensed an inward racing going on. I knew he was always deep in thought and always thinking about the future, financial ventures, and projects on which he was working. I approached Craig about the lack of congruency I sensed between his surface calm and his racing mind. I asked him if he had ever given thought to the fact that he might have been an undiagnosed hyperactive child who had learned to settle down the best he could on his own. Not surprisingly he said "yes!" We explored this together.

Once I realized what was happening, I was able to work with and around it very well. Up until that time, I would experience a lack of Peace because of Craig's continual focus on the future. I allowed it to take me out of experiencing the joy of "the Moment." Craig was wired differently than me. However, his energy seemed to dominate our interactions.

Craig lived in another state, and when I would go to his home, he would pack many activities into my allotted time. I am sure he just wanted me to get to know his world, and I was happy to do that. Yet, I would have just settled into experiencing "the Moment" or the person he had introduced me to when he would whisk me off to the next activity. I approached Craig about my need to slow down and be "in the Moment." He agreed to try it himself, yet this was extremely difficult for him.

I offered Craig an opportunity to see what I was talking about. I asked him to sit on the couch with me for 10 minutes and do nothing, just sit on the couch and be in "the Moment." He said, "that's not a problem; in fact I'm tired and can use the rest." Because of my past experiences with Craig, I didn't think he would be able to sit still, even if he needed the rest. After approximately three minutes, I felt that he was restless. We had been sitting in quiet during this time, but I sensed that he needed to talk. I said "is something wrong?" He said "Don't let me forget to call Kenneth about wiring the money to Phoenix. It is important that I do it by 3:00". I agreed, but his restlessness increased. I told him to make the call, so that he could relax. He made the phone call, but then came back and acknowledged his inability to be "in the Moment".

Craig and I never had a handle on what was really going on until we labeled the problem as possibly the result of an adult version of his childhood hyperactivity. We made great progress in this area: Craig had more experiences of "being in the Moment," and I was able to assure that I never let his focus on the future rob my Peace or my ability to stay "in the Moment."

There is another related concept that can interfere with your ability to be "in the Moment," if you allow it. It is another form of missing "the Moment," Most people have multiple roles (parent, employee, citizen, spouse, friend, etc.) You need to become conscious of the fact that if you take on too many roles, or do not allow yourself to fully experience each role, you may feel ineffectiveness in your roles, and be unable to be in "the Moment".

I will use the nursing profession, since it is the one with which I am most familiar. Nursing is very intense, and nurses are constantly dealing with crisis and emotional issues of patients, so to be effective they must be very engaged and focused. Many nurses are also parents. For the purpose of illustration, let's say you are a nurse, and your child had a fever before you left for work. Your baby sitter has never cared for your child during an illness before. Your mind keeps drifting back to home. Many nurses will struggle through such challenges throughout a shift. They are not physically at home, they are not emotionally at work, and they are not "in the Moment."

In my former role as a nursing administrator and my current role as an instructor, I always recommend that practitioners ask another nurse or student to provide care to their patients while they call home and talk to the baby sitter. I suggest they become totally focused on the child during the phone conversation, not thinking about their patients, as they are adequately covered by another nurse. Once practitioners have come to Peace and some resolution of their dilemma, they can let it go for a while. This strategy allows them to return to their patients with the energy, focus, and level of engagement their patients deserve; they feel more at Peace and are more effective in both their professional and parental roles.

The reason I am focusing on this topic is because of a question that many of my students have asked me. They often express a desire for Peace, but they don't think it is possible with their hectic schedules. One student in particular asked that I specifically address the "hurried life." I welcomed the opportunity, because it conjures up such a clear picture.

The hurried life is one that many people, unfortunately, experience and live. I can just imagine this person who rushes from activity to activity, and rushes between activities, not even enjoying the car ride between activities. I envision this person as a woman, but the situation equally relates to men. I see the woman:

- hurriedly picking the children up at school and quickly asking about homework
- realizing she forgot needed sports equipment for her son's football practice
- not having enough gas in the car, then stopping for gas and putting the family behind schedule
- running back home for the sports equipment
- talking on the cell phone to her husband to make sure he picks up the milk and bread and will be able to pick up their other child from guitar lessons
- while at football practice, writing out the grocery list and figuring out when to stop at the library for a child's book that is needed for a future assignment
- preparing for what she will do at the computer that night to finish up the work she did not do while at work (because she probably

called her husband several times during the day or spent time thinking about their busy evening)

and so on, and so on, and so on! And we haven't even talked about dinner, homework, showers, opening the mail, and the laundry yet!

You can almost feel the stress just thinking about this woman's life! A little analogy here might help address the feeling that people have when they say they "have too much on their plate." I have always recommended a different picture. I agree that the picture of "too much on a plate" is not a healthy concept. It is better to think of it as many plates, with one thing on each plate. Many plates are easier to deal with. If everything is lumped onto one plate, it is overwhelming before you even begin. You would probably even have trouble figuring out *where* to begin. However, if there is one thing on each plate, you deal totally with the plate that is in front of you. It is easy to figure out how to get started and what needs to be done. When that plate is clear, you move on to the next plate. The picture of addressing one plate at a time is more manageable. This leads to the next issue, that of looking at how many plates you have.

A helpful way of thinking about this issue is to think of the man at the talent show who spins plates on top of sticks. At first, when he spins one plate, he feels good. As he gets three or four plates spinning, he begins to feel more accomplished and better about himself. He feels so good that he begins spinning more and more, until he eventually gets to the point where he cannot keep all of the plates spinning. He runs back and forth trying to keep all of the plates in the air. The more he tries and the faster he goes, the more frantic he becomes and the less effective he is as a plate spinner. Possibly, he added one more plate than he should have. One falls and breaks, then the next. He feels deflated and like a failure. He might have had 16 plates spinning, but he focuses on the one that caused the whole act to flop.

See any similarities to life? I am not opposed to filling up your life with things you choose, as long as it is a conscious choice.

And not all of the things you choose have to be productive or highly active. You may choose to read one hour a day or watch a movie. I always have enough time to do everything I want to do, because I am highly conscious that how I spend my time is my choice at all times. Even when something by its nature requires my time, I look at the whole picture and determine what could be given up so that I feel a sense of Peace and unhurriedness in the rest of my life.

There is a tendency to fall victim to the feeling that we have to do it all. However, in the process, we don't do any of it well. And we never have the opportunity to really experience the things we think we are choosing to be included in our lives. We simply rush from activity to activity, and usually during any activity, we are focusing on getting to the next one or next three. Life is what happens while you are busy making plans.

I always monitor how much I have going on in my life at any given time. I have always had the philosophy that if I am going to do anything, I am going to do it well and with 100% effort and attention. If I can't give it 100%, I need to put it off and come back to it when I can do it the way I want and that feels good for me. This philosophy has allowed me to enjoy all of my roles, feel effective, and have a sense of Peace and joy as I experience life while serving in a variety of roles.

One example of taking charge of how much I include in my life happened last night. As previously mentioned, I am on the Zoning Board of Appeals in my town. It has been very rewarding and a real education and growth experience for me. I have given it my all. However, as this book nears publication, I have needed to evaluate, if I can afford to have several of my Thursday evenings devoted to my role as a Board member. I certainly have a passion about protecting the rural, small town nature of my community. This is important to me. Yet, I made the choice to resign from the Board, with hopes of returning to it in the future when my schedule permits.

My family knows of the dilemma I face as this book is released. I enjoy my current roles and the pace of my life. From the depths of my soul, I know how important the concept of Peace management is, and I truly wish that every person who wanted it could have access to Peace management. However, I would not want this book to take on a life of its own and change my life in directions that I am not ready or willing to incorporate. I will have to practice what I preach, making certain that I am doing the concept of Peace management justice, while maintaining a balance with my personal life and my other roles.

I have a radar of sorts that lets me know when I approach "spinning one too many plates." Even though the decision to eliminate a plate is often difficult, I am very clear that the results pay off well. This allows more time to be "in the Moment" as I experience the rest of life, which ultimately allows Peace.

Being a wife is a role I take very seriously. My husband and I have very full lives, what some might call busy. But I never see it that way. In fact, people say to me "oh, you are so busy." I kindly deny it and state, "no, I am doing everything I want to be doing and nothing that I don't want to be doing. My life is filled appropriately." The word "busy" is what I reserve for people who unintentionally, or without analyzing activities in relation to the whole picture, fill up their schedules with *too many* things.

I have seven items on my "to do" list for today, all things I consciously choose and want in my life. Yet, despite the fact that there were a number of things on my list, this morning my husband and I took a half hour to sit outside and have coffee before we began our day. This satisfied my need as a wife for the time being. I supported my husband in his ideas and plans for the day, as he supported me with my plans. We threw around some possibilities of how we would like to spend the latter part or our evening together after we had accomplished what we were about to do. We were both totally "in the Moment" when we were having coffee, enjoying our time together. When we realized we were beginning to give actual thought to how we were going to proceed in our day, we realized it was probably time to move on.

The second main reason that people do not experience "the Moment" is because of the negative emotions they experience related to thoughts of the past or future. Let's explore this concept. Given that we live in a world that has embraced the concept of time, we need to understand what that really means. This will be somewhat difficult. Even the great thinkers and philosophers have grappled with the concept of time as a reality. Therefore, we will just pull out what we need in relation to its impact on Peace.

Does time exist? Well, in the way that we think of it in this world, I guess the answer would be "yes." We tend to think of time in a very linear way; there was something before this, and there is now, and there will be something after this. Another way of saying this is *there is past, present, and future.*

Let me challenge you here (and I am aware that I am getting a little deep). I said there *was* something before this, there *is* now, and there *will be* something after this. Anyone who has taken a foreign language course or an English grammar course knows that these words are conjugations of the verb "to be." So even in concept, this is confusing. The infinitive "to be" itself gives the impression that there is only the present. To "be" cannot happen in the past or the future, you can only "be" in the present. When you were "be-ing" in the past, that was an accurate use of that verb at that time. But as soon as you are beyond that experience, it is no longer possible to "be" there. Okay, take a moment here. Don't read any more yet. Let this one sink in.

* * *

So, if the present is the only place you could really "be," and it is also the only thing that really *exists*, then how do we interpret these concepts that we call the "past" and the "future"? (This is very important if you are trying to take Peace management to the next level, so make sure you take the time to get this.) When I am in the present, the only place I can really *be*, this is reality. This is existing and experiencing. There can be no negative emotions in the Now! Okay, I know you are thinking. "what the heck is she talking about?"

Hang with me here. I am a teacher by profession, I will make sure you get it before I move on.

The past and future are only thoughts. I don't even want to say that they are the experiences from your thoughts, because that gives them too much credit and it's not the truth. The past *happens* in your mind *only*. And, you are the only one who experiences your past; no one else can. Other people who shared the same experience with you can also have thoughts of that past, but those thoughts are *their* thoughts. They may attach some significance and meaning to the thoughts. The significance and meaning they attach may be similar to yours or vastly different. No matter what, they are still only thoughts. Doesn't that fact, in and of itself, allow you to minimize the effects that your past creates for you?

That dinner party you went to last month, where you said some things that created resentment by your sister-in-law and caused you much subsequent anguish—well, any feelings you are having about it now are only because of your thoughts; the emotions result from those thoughts. Whenever the "past" comes up for you, it is a thought. If you are having a negative emotion, it is because of the thought. The emotion doesn't just jump up by itself. It is attached to the thought. Without the thought, there is no emotion.

And if your sister-in-law is still having negative emotions because of that conversation, remember, that is her issue, not your issue. Get her a copy of this book and let her do her own work on this one.

If you will remember from an earlier technique: nothing is inherently bad or good, it is only perceived that way because of the meaning that we attach to it. That is a large part of what our past is, events embellished with the meaning we give to it.

A great example of this occurred to me recently. I had a dream that a car pulled up in my driveway in the middle of the night. Two teenage boys and a teenage girl got out and were walking around in my yard, obviously up to no good. In my dream, I asked my husband to wake up and get his gun. Soon after that, I woke up. My heart was racing; I was sweating and breathing fast. I had a charge from a "night thought." It was all in my thoughts! Nothing had really happened. The charge resulted from a thought that was not even based on an actual event.

The future, as far as being a thought, is even less significant than the past. At least in the past, something definitely did happen. Our fearful thoughts of the future, are only abstract possibilities that are a sum total of our life experiences and worries, projected onto something that is only a possibility. We give a great deal of time and attention in our thoughts to something that is a thought, and nothing more. Are we messed up, or what?

I actually had an experience this morning, demonstrating very clearly to me how giving excess thought to something in the future is often a waste of time. I have been receiving several unsolicited faxes from a stock brokerage company. I received one overnight which used the last piece of paper in the fax machine. I thought it was time to put an end to this.

I decided to call the company. I anticipated a lengthy conversation and that I would probably have to talk to many people to get my name removed from their list. I spent a great deal of time thinking about the best strategy, then I called the number. What I got immediately was a recording telling me what to do if I wanted to remove my name from the fax list. I was done in 20 seconds and never had to talk to a single person to get this problem resolved. I chuckled as I walked away from the phone. I love to laugh at myself.

Negative emotions are always caused by thoughts which are related to the past or the future. The following example shows that even in what you might consider an extreme case of experiencing the emotion of fear, the emotion results from letting in thoughts of the past or future. Fear is the *emotion* we feel when we sense our current existence is jeopardized.

If you were working in a bank and someone pulled out a gun and pointed it at your head, you would feel fear. This is a natural response because of what you associate with such a situation. You would be afraid of being shot, and you know being shot would probably cause serious injury or death (because you learned about it in school or from TV or somewhere else). The fear you would feel in that instance might cause you to react properly, in a self-preserving way. So, I am not saying the emotion of fear at a moment requiring a fight or flight response is detrimental. It serves you well in these instances.

The emotion of fear occurs because of your association with past thoughts or future fears. It's just that, in these type of examples, the fear takes root in a fraction of a second. If you are not clear here, possibly this unusual example may illustrate this response better. Imagine you are an alien dropped onto Earth and your job is to work at a bank. On your planet, when you meet someone new, you hold up a gun-like apparatus to the other person's head. This gives the other person love and positive energy. Therefore, if the robber from the first example held a gun up to your head, you would have no negative thoughts from your past and no fear of the future. In your mind, nothing bad comes from guns, only love and positive energy.

I know this is a bizarre example, but I am trying to illustrate that we experience any emotion, even those to which we do not give highly conscious attention, because of a thought. In the fight/flight response it happens quickly, because it is a flash thought of our past or future. The negative emotion is not about the actual experience.

Let's apply the concepts of past, present, and future to Peace. There is Peace in "the Moment," no negative emotion. Whenever you are removed from the Peace of "the Moment," step back and look at it. It is always caused by some thought of the past or future. You don't give thought to or about the Now, *you only experience* the Now. It is impossible to think about the Now. You may think *in* the Now, but not *about* the Now. Even good or pleasant thoughts take you out of the experience and into judging or comparing. It might be a lovely day, but as soon as you think that, it leads you into the thought mode. This will probably also start a whole chain of other thoughts.

You may be having pleasant thoughts or business-type thoughts. This could be a very enjoyable time. For example, you may be experiencing the joy of planning, exploring a concept, remembering something, or making a mental note of something. It is thought on a more conscious level, as if you are choosing to think about these things at this time. This is a form of the Now; you are experiencing the current "Moment." However, as soon as any negative emotions enter, you are no longer experiencing the Now.

Applying this concept of experiencing the Now is how we can learn to live life "in the Moment" and experience a higher level of joy and Peace. Essentially, the goal is to work toward not having any more thoughts of the past and future that create negative emotions for you. Have you heard the advice to take "one day at a time"? That task actually seems a bit overwhelming for me. It is easier to think "one Moment at a time." I can do this! And if I truly strive to experience the Now, one Moment at a time, it eventually becomes my *continual Now, or the way I live*.

* * * What it is, of sorts, is

an immediate Now + an immediate Now + an immediate Now . . .

this will eventually lead to the experience of
living "in the Moment".

Expand the "instant Now" to be the
"experiencing Now".

Think of some of the most pleasant and joyful experiences you have had recently. This past Sunday, my family had a barbecue at our home. On Monday, my mother called to tell me that it was such a wonderful day: peaceful, joyful, and loving. I helped her to realize it was because we all remained "in the Now" most of the day, only allowing our focus to be on experiencing "the Moment". I never left “the Moment” the whole day. I think part of my mother’s experience was feeling that energy.

My mother has recently experienced a number of losses by death in a very short period of time. She lost her mother, father, best friend, and a cousin. She has had difficulty with Peace and staying “in the Now,” but she is making great strides in this area. Her awareness of the benefit of being “in the Now” on Sunday will certainly be an impetus to get her back on track.

Recently, we were at a restaurant with my family. We found a place that offered inexpensive lobster tails. Even that was part of the fun. We were enjoying “the Moment,” the company, and life in general. My father, trying to protect his family, in a very fatherly way began sharing a story about something he had read in the paper or heard on TV. He began to relay the story of a woman who was selling a car and opened her garage door and . . . . I can’t even share any more details of the story with you because that is as far as I let the story progress.

I told my father that I didn’t want to let any fear-based thoughts enter my consciousness. I asked him not to share any more of that story. I caught him off guard initially. But within moments, we were back to laughing and continuing with the wonderful experience. When I am experiencing fear related to a thought, I am no longer “in the Moment.”

My own history and direct exposure to the tragedy of others has created plenty of potential fears for me. I don’t need anything else to enter my consciousness. I have done fine with my own list of fears. Plus, my family has done what most families do. They want to help their loved ones to avoid any unnecessary bad experiences, so they willingly pass on their fears and concerns from their past experiences or knowledge. No harm is ever intended. In fact, good is intended. But hearing about bad experiences certainly overloads your consciousness with thoughts of the past and fears about the possibilities in the future. And that is not good!

I attempt to withhold passing any of my fears to my son. Like me, he is doing fine creating his own list. I know some will disagree with this parenting approach, and I understand. In fact, I know I do pass some fears on to him (like my fears of big, bad dogs and drunk drivers). But I would rather spend the time teaching my son to listen to his gut and make his own decisions. He has become very skilled at this. There is no possible way that I could think of every situation in which he should react with avoidance. He needs to be able to decide on his own.

As a parent, you will want to give advice to your children. For example, you may need to inform them that is unwise to walk on a frozen lake in the winter. You can do this in a very non-fear based way. In fact, that is the most healthy way and can actually be used as a way to teach your children to be better decision makers. If you tell them the horror stories where kids knowingly risked walking on a frozen pond, fell in, and drowned, your children may someday see walking on ice as a challenge. Thinking as children do, they may want to prove to themselves that there is a way to walk on ice successfully or that falling through the ice won't happen to them.

Rather than scaring your children, when talking to them as you see a frozen lake, you may ask "do you think it would be a good idea to walk across that lake? What could happen?" Explore the whole concept with the child and allow them to come up with their own conclusions, under your guidance. The choice to walk on ice will be internalized more as a *bad decision* if your children make that decision on their own, rather than receiving the fear/quasi-challenge from you. It is all about the manner or style that you choose to educate your children.

A current issue I am dealing with is helping my son as he tries to make a decision about playing football. He is a very good baseball player with dreams of playing major league ball. He has some interest in playing football. I have discussed the choice with him, making sure he is aware of the need to protect his body from injury if he wants to play major league caliber ball. He would need to have all his body parts in good working order.

Although my son thinks I have placed my fear in him, I have not. In fact, my *placing* a fear in him is impossible, but back to the story. My son could not have picked up any fear from me, as I have no fear about injuries. I can deal with the broken bones and the need for stitches. I'm a nurse. I think what he is actually reflecting on is his own decision making process.

Yes, I may have placed awareness of the potential consequences of playing football in my son's mind, but I did not do it from a place of fear. He has interpreted the risk of injury as a major consideration in his decision. Any tendency to choose not to play football in his mind is based on fear of injury and its impact on playing baseball, and that idea was initiated by me. So he associates the fear with me. Anyway, I don't even see his thought of injury while playing football as a fear, as fear being a negative *emotion*. There is no imminent danger. He is not even playing football at this time. Fear will be differentiated from anxiety and worry in the technique called "Eliminate the Fear". What he is experiencing is simply part of the decision making process. In fact, he has no charge when he is talking about the fear. It is simply a consideration he is taking into account.

However, if my son was playing football, and during the game he was experiencing a charge related to a possible imminent injury, that would be a fear. It would take him out of "the Moment" of playing football and into fearful thoughts about future possibilities.

My husband requests I put a disclaimer or qualifier here, so, for him . . . if you need to place fears in your children, you have my blessing, they are your children.

I don't want to present myself or my goal as naive or ignorant. Fear will pop into my existence when it will serve me well. When the situation necessitates, fear will mobilize me to react. However, I don't want it to enter my thoughts at a time when it is not necessary or relevant to what is going on in the immediate situation. When this happens, Peace is lost. Fear is a negative emotion that comes from either regrets from the past that are projected onto the future or general fears of the future, and both rob your Now/Peace. Remember, none of these situations exist in the Now. As soon as negative emotions enter, you are in thoughts about the past or future, not experiencing "the Now."

Fear should not be confused with caution. Fear is the emotion, caution is part of the thought process when making a decision. No emotion is associated with caution. I may use caution not to walk near men cutting down trees. It would be fear if a large tree limb were falling my way. Both the use of caution and fear in this example (causing you to run from the falling limb) would serve you well. Sitting in your office, having fear of the dangers of a falling limb at home during an electrical storm would not serve you or your health well. This type of fear is more closely associated with fret or worry.

Although not all of our thoughts are laden with emotion, many are. Earlier, I had mentioned a different type of thinking. I called this the business mode. It is when we are engaged in very purposeful thinking and planning. You can actually be "in the Moment" when you are engaged in this type of thinking. I know this may initially seem to contradict all I have said to this point, but it doesn't.

When I am in business mode of thinking, I am definitely "in the Moment." I enjoy planning and working on lectures. I might be remembering something I learned in the past or thinking of how to present something in the future. I am thinking non-stop. But I am in my element, my "Now." This can apply to any purposeful thinking. If, however, I notice some type of negative emotion come into play, it is my radar that I am no longer "in the Now." I have let some past or future concern enter my "Moment." I might be working on a lecture about kidney failure. This may spark memories of my friend who died recently. He had a medical condition that caused him to be very worried about going into kidney failure before he died. My mind and thoughts might swirl down and I might become consumed with various negative thoughts and emotions. When negative emotions enter, I need to be aware that I am no longer "in the Moment." In the case above, I was thinking about the past.

If I am working on a lecture about the electrical system of the heart and resulting rhythm disturbances, I might feel a concern about any potential lack of prior education and experience my students might have in this area. This thought soon turns to a form of worry of "how will I catch them up quickly so I can cover the more complex topics?" Can you see that I let fears of the future take me out of the Now? And you know what, I usually find that my students have very strong education backgrounds, so I never have to address these concerns anyway. What I have since started to do in this and similar instances is create a back up plan from the start, avoiding any perceived need for worry.

One final very important related concept is shielding yourself from the negative energy of others. Earlier, I focused on the explanation of Craig's difficulty with staying "in the Moment." I enjoy living "in the Moment", yet I picked up on Craig's energy. In a sense, part of my issue was subconscious thoughts related to past experiences of being pulled out of "the Moment" when I was with Craig. However, I am sure that his energy transferred to me, giving me an unsettled feeling, or loss of Peace. I am sure that some of my discomfort was direct internalization of Craig's energy. His sense of impatience and future orientation created a rushed approach to our shared experiences.

Therefore, again I suggest analyzing any time or pattern that feels unsettled or lacking Peace. You may be amazed at what you find on your own explorations! This concept of taking on the energy of others is very complex. Simply bring an awareness to this issue. Think back to a time you attended a comedy club, a sporting event, a wedding, a funeral (where you might not have even know the deceased), or any similar activity. Did the mood or energy of the crowd have any direct effect on you?

In summary, I want to reiterate that I am not suggesting that we do not need to plan or give thought to the future or the past. The difference is that the past and future should not be the place from which we experience life. If you find yourself frequently having negative emotions, stress, or a charge, admit to yourself that it is the way you are *experiencing* life. In a way, it is the flavor you taste or the color of the glasses you are choosing to wear as you experience your life. It affects all facets of the way you experience life.

Your focus should be on experiencing life from a place of Peace or joy. Those are the natural emotions tied to "the Now" or "the Moment." When we experience a negative emotion, it is because we are living or experiencing in the past or future, which is not an experience at all. It is just a thought that is causing us to have that particular experience. The only place you can choose Peace is in the present. You cannot chose Peace in the past or future.

I apologize for any confusion I might have created as you worked through these abstract concepts, or if I lost you at times. If you were willing to genuinely "be with this" during your reading, you took away exactly what you needed for this time. You may want to re-read this section in six months and see if anything else applies to you, allowing you to relate more of this discussion of "the Moment" to your life, path, and growth.

The attached exercise will allow you to increase awareness of your frequent removals from "the Moment" or Peace.

Exercise (AA):

Peace in the Moment

Goals for this section:

- Identify the link between feeling a charge and its relationship to thoughts about the past or the future
- List all your roles and activities and label each of them as one of your spinning plates
- Decide whether your life is adequately filled with things you consciously choose to have in your life
- Bring an awareness to moments when you are experiencing a charge about one thing, while you are doing something else
- Set up a plan which will allow you to get back to "the Moment"
- Experience the ability to be in a quiet (not meditative) state and fully experience "the Moment"
- Expand the immediate Now into the experiencing Now
- Become aware of your direct uptake of the negative energy radiating from another person

---

Activity A:

The next time you become aware that you have a charge, STOP in your tracks. What caused the charge? Identify what thoughts of the past or thoughts of the future gave you that charge.

Once your identify the thought, tell yourself "there is no value in tearing down my health. I release the thought." THEN *RELEASE* IT!

Activity B:

I am sure you will need a separate sheet of paper for this exercise. So, go get it. Yeah, now! Go get it.

Make two columns:

- In one column, write down all of your roles (mom, dad, employee, sister, son, neighbor, PTA member, etc.)
- In the second column write down all the things you do (homework with your children—and list it separately for each child, drive the kids to religion class, grocery shop, pick up prescriptions for you mother, cancer fund raising, doing the laundry, cleaning the house, walking the dog, cleaning the hamster cage, etc.)

Do you see where I am going?

Now, if you want to have a little fun, get a poster size piece of paper and draw several ovals, representing plates. Draw a stick under each plate. Put one of your roles and activities inside each plate. How many plates do you have spinning? 600?

So next time you decide to add something else to your life, or better yet, next time someone else asks you to do something else, ask them to fill in another plate and stick it on your poster.

Now the hard part. Do you want to hang on to all of those activities and roles in your life? If the answer is "no," then start your plan. I realize some things you can't give up, no matter how much you would like to (like paying your bills), but just about everything else could be changed, negotiated, or given up.

And stop saying I am not realistic. That will only keep you in your rut. You can stay there if you want, but then stop complaining about it. I am living proof that plates can be eliminated. I constantly change which plates I have in the air. So do the people I counsel, and with much reported success.

You might say something like, "I can't give up school." I say you *can* but *don't*. It is your choice to be there. That is one of the plates you are deciding to keep in the air.

Just one final question. Did any of your plates include things that you consider fun or relaxing? Does that give you any more insight into how your life is filled up?

Activity C:

If you experience a charge, stop and analyze it. Is your thought, which takes you out of "the Moment," in regard to something going on at the same time as your current activity? A sick child? Results from a lab test you are expecting today? If so, is it possible to take care of that matter now, so that you can go back to your current activity with full attention and enjoyment?

Activity D:

This exercise will give you an accurate taste of what it feels like to be in "the Moment."

After you read the rest of this section, put the book down. Sit in the room and just *be*. I am not talking about meditating. Keep your eyes open. Remain in a very alert state. Look at all the things in the room. Notice the colors, the sounds, the temperature of the room—but do not make any judgments about them or have any thoughts.

Don't think "I need to clean that table" or "there are so many papers." Simply look at them. Move on to looking at the next thing. If you find yourself getting distracted, become aware of your breathing, then return to looking at the room contents and becoming aware of your surroundings. Do this exercise for 5 minutes.

Activity E:

Practice expanding the immediate Now into the experiencing Now.

Go make a piece of toast. Be aware of the cool feel of the air as you open the refrigerator and the smell of the bread as you take it out of its packaging. Feel the texture of the bread as you hold it. Become aware of the pressure you exert as you push the lever on the toaster. Which small muscles tightened as you performed this? Smell the bread toasting. Butter a portion of the bread, and listen to the crunching sound. Put jelly on the remainder of the toast. Sit down. Feel the chair and be aware of your posture. Taste the buttered toast, then the jellied toast. How does it feel in your mouth? Be aware of the muscles during chewing. Listen to the sound as you chew. Be aware of your throat region as you swallow.

Then keep your awareness on your movement as you walk back to the room where you were. Feel your feet hitting the floor, or the cushion under the carpet. This is the experiencing Now. No negative emotions, no thoughts of past or future. Only a feeling of Peace.

Now, begin applying experiencing "the Moment" to the life you live.

Activity F:

Develop an awareness of how your energy might change depending on the people with whom you are interacting.

People may not appear to have an overt positive or negative energy, but if you watch the changes in yourself when you are in someone else's presence, you will probably begin to understand their energy and how you are internalizing it.

Once you become aware of your reaction to other people, you will need to realize that it is not always possible to keep yourself away from people who carry negative energy. But you can bring your awareness to your interactions and make a decision not to pick up or take on their energy.

If you want to take this strategy one step further, see if your genuine Peace can change the energy of the person who is radiating negativity. You will be amazed at the results. Remember, others will pick up your energy, just as you may pick up theirs. If you remain at Peace, you will have a calming effect on others and the situation.

Technique: You are Hurt By Your Anger

Anger is so prevalent in our society and it is a very potent thief of Peace. Not only does anger harm our emotional well-being and Peace, but research is beginning to demonstrate a greater link between anger and health problems. Anger and hate are probably two of the most negative emotions we have.

There are two terms we usually use in relation to this emotion: rage and anger. There is a difference. Rage is the intense manifestation of anger during the fight or flight response. Anger is the low level emotion habitually carried with a person. Better explained, anger is like the *simmering* emotion and rage is the full blown *boil* of the emotion.

Rage is what is felt and manifested during the adrenaline-rush, fight or flight response of anger. This rage is easily called upon in a person who is already simmering with low level anger. Anger is the form of this emotion that is continuously present and hidden just below the surface in some individuals.

It would be very difficult to eradicate the intense anger (rage) without first dealing with the low level anger. The goal is to become a person who experiences Peace as the predominant state of being through becoming a very successful Peace manager. This goal is made in an effort to change your essence, in an attempt to ban anger and the resulting rage.

Anger and rage are manifested even in children, usually borne out of frustration. As we age and mature, we often take the first step, which is developing more sophisticated ways of dealing with frustration. But it should not stop there. We need to change our essence to one of Peace, which then abolishes the feeling of frustration. This step is what moves individuals away from the potential of experiencing rage. We need to *get this*, get it *deeply*, and get it *now*. It is very harmful to us!

Two very common destructive forms of anger are now household words: road rage and domestic violence. Other drivers and partners are easy outlets for rage in a person who carries anger. Unfortunately, a lack of internal control and power prompts an individual with anger to release it in what they perceive as safe environments. Those safe areas are family members who have a known love for you and strangers whom you will never see again after the episode on the road.

Yes, your anger does hurt others around you, and I do care about the people who end up being a victim of someone else's anger. However, by this point in the book, you should be aware that they are responsible for their own management of Peace and life situations. What I wish to emphasize is that ***YOU*** are hurt by your anger.

The harmful chemicals that your body releases during low levels of stress as well as intense stress (fight or flight) are essentially the same chemicals your body releases during low levels and intense periods of anger. These chemicals create all the subsequent cellular and molecular changes that have a negative impact on your health.

Rage rears its ugly head easily, with relatively little prompting in a person who carries that low-level simmering of anger. Therefore, by gradually implementing the strategies of Peace management to the point where you change your essence, your anger will disappear, along with the tendency to experience rage. For example, think of the most genuinely calm, serene person you know. Can you imagine this person being prompted to the point of severe rage? Probably not.

Some strategies will work better than others for both promoting Peace and eliminating anger. There are several presented in this book, but to get the greatest impact, you must be willing to create your own strategies for maintaining Peace and make this process your own. This "Peace-full" state will allow you to get to the point where you become aware that *there is no place for anger*.

Road rage has been an unmanageable problem for many. You need to implement any strategy in the beginning to start eliminating it. I often suggest even artificial-seeming strategies in the initial stages, simply to get the process started. For example, when a person cuts you off, you can imagine that they were just diagnosed with cancer and are very distracted. In a twisted way, this strategy promotes compassion.

My father knows I have worked with many people on overcoming road rage and have taught the strategy described above. He called this morning to tell me he was sending me an article from the newspaper in Florida. The article noted that a man had been driving and was cut off by a woman. He was so angry that he followed her to her home. When she got out of her car, he began shouting at her. She quickly cut him off with an apology and said, "I'm sorry. I just left my doctor's office and was told that I have a brain tumor." Fact *is* stranger than fiction.

I recently ran into someone whom I worked with years ago. I told him about Peace management. He said this was very much needed in his workplace. He works in a hospital department made up entirely of men. He told of the incompetence that runs rampant in his department. He said the department is a breeding ground for anger, yet it is not socially acceptable to manifest anger in the work setting. Therefore, he said many men are having marital troubles, because they are taking out their anger on their wives and kids. They all said they feel very unsettled and guilty for their "child-like" reactions. So again, these men are not only hurting their families, they are hurting themselves.

Become aware of any rage you experience. Determine if you carry a low level of anger. As Peace becomes "the way you are" you will not even need strategies. Anger and Peace cannot coexist as your essence, *and* rage and Peace cannot coexist as your experience of a situation. The choice is yours!

Exercise (BB):

You Are Hurt by your Anger

Goals for this section:

- Analyze any possible rage reactions you may have
- Identify the correlation between rage and an underlying anger
- Identify how past anger has hurt you
- Outline strategies to assist you with replacing anger with Peace
- Analyze any reduction in underlying anger that you have already experienced as a result of implementing Peace management

---

Activity A:

Think back over the past month or so. Did you have any outbursts where you either screamed or reacted in a physical way (punching a pillow, throwing something, trying to drive another car off the road, slamming a door)? Would you say the feeling at the time was rage?

Were the episodes of rage representative of your normal pattern of reacting? Did they occur at a times when you were experiencing anger in relation to another event or person that was not involved in the rage episode? Do you think you displaced anger but projected it onto a safer moment or person?

Activity B:

Have you ever experienced an illness or injury during or immediately following a period of intense anger or rage?

Have you ever felt guilt, shame, or remorse after exhibiting rage?

Do you see any benefit in anger? Be honest. If you see a benefit, what is it? Is it worth the loss of Peace and the resulting physical harm?

Do you want to release anger and replace it with Peace?

Activity C:

Sit in quiet for a moment. Think about the things that provoke anger and rage in you. Develop a very concrete plan for not allowing yourself to experience anger. Try techniques like "Go There," "Cultivate Compassion," "Still the Mind," or any other creative avenue.

Continually monitor yourself for growth in this area. Anger reduction requires intense desire and work. Acknowledge any prior growth you have had in this area. Give attention to what it is that is working for you, and devote more energy to this approach.

Technique: Eliminate the Fear

People often ask me "how can I get rid of the fear I have?" The way most people address fear, is like putting the cart before the horse. You cannot fix your emotions about the future without first fixing what is going on in the present. That is why, although fear is so prevalent, it was not presented earlier in the book. It is not a quick fix, nor does it simply involve a will to turn it off. You must first achieve a sense of Peace before fear will vanish from your existence.

You can always instantly abolish a single fear thought by simply choosing to eliminate it, but fear is usually very insidious. It becomes a part of your existence. The best way to change your thought patterns about the future is to change the way you are in the present. Many have fear when they think about the future. That is because it is a mirror, or better yet, a projection, of our current state on to the future. The only way to release fear about the future is to have better experiences in the present.

How do you do that? Well, all the strategies and techniques in this book are intended to eventually change your essence to one who experiences Peace on a regular, if not continual basis. But let's focus on an easy target for things that rob your Peace in the present. Don't let the past taint your present. You cannot change the occurrences of the past, simply your thoughts about them. If you release the thoughts that cause the negative emotions associated with the past, for example, regret, shame, or guilt, you will release the stress in the present. Remember, stress replaces Peace. Any negative emotion robs your Peace. So, if you can eliminate the negative emotions associated with your past, you will have Peace in the present. If you have Peace in the present, there will not be any room for the negative emotions associated with the future, such as fear, worry, and anxiety.

Differentiating fear, worry and anxiety is only necessary for understanding the terminology. All will be treated similarly with

Peace management. All three terms relate to thoughts projected on to the future that manifest as a negative emotion. Fear can either be used as a catch-all term for these future concerns or it could be used to distinguish a concept from the concepts of anxiety and worry.

When the terms are used to differentiate one from another, fear is generally used to describe the emotion when danger is imminent. There is something occurring at present that creates a thought which then creates the emotion. Anxiety or worry are used when no imminent danger exists at present but thoughts create concern for future possibilities.

People often have the most trouble at the end of the day. Your night thoughts (right before sleep, which probably keep you awake beyond your desire) and your dreams (which can cause anxiety) are simply a reflection or extension of your day thoughts. The best strategy for changing these fear-provoking or anxiety-provoking night thoughts is to change your day thoughts.

There is a spiral effect that occurs. Your thoughts reflect who you are, and who you are is reflected in your thoughts. It is much easier to change the direction of the spiral by changing your thoughts. You are always creating the new you. What you can improve at the conscious level will improve you at the subconscious level. Who you are at the moment creates the type of thoughts you have, and the type of thoughts that you have create the current you.

If you have thoughts of fear in the present, you create a fearful you. The "fearful you" creates more fear thoughts. More fear thoughts create a more fearful you. And so on . . .

I have one student who very bravely told her story on how her continual fear thoughts played out in her reality. Lauren said she was always a "what if?" kid. She said she actually fatigued her Mom by always thinking the worst, having fear, and saying "yeah, but what if . . ." Well as fate had it, she experienced a tremendous amount of turbulence in her life, all in a period of months. Many of her "what ifs" came true. Her family home burned down, and her pets perished in the fire. Two weeks after she began dating her boyfriend, his sister drowned. Her grandmother developed cancer and died. Plus, there were many more, relatively minor disasters.

These disasters perpetuated Lauren's "what if" thinking. This thought pattern became more of who she was. She tried desperately to deal with this burdensome thinking as she felt she was in the downward spiral. She was very clear that it was harmful to her and that her thoughts about unwanted possibilities did not prevent them from occurring. She realized her fear thoughts served no purpose and were all-consuming. It wasn't until she began Peace management, that she realized she had to change her essence in order to achieve Peace and release the fear. She admits that she has a long way to go, but feels that she is on the right path, she is spiraling up, and is never turning back.

I have a personal example of how my essence abolished my fear thoughts. Several years ago, when my son was a baby, my husband stopped to offer assistance at a car accident. The car in question had almost run us off the road, but then drifted down into a nearby parking lot. When we went up to the car, we noticed the driver was slumped over. He was not breathing and did not have a pulse. No one else in the area knew the man or knew CPR. I did CPR by myself, including mouth-to-mouth resuscitation. The man was resuscitated, but later that night died at the hospital. I found out more about him.

I found out that the victim's son had recently died of AIDS, and his obituary stated that he had recently been treated for a viral infection. I didn't know if that virus was HIV or not. I did some investigating. I found out, that the recent virus had been a simple upper respiratory infection. Yet I still did not know if the man *also* had the AIDS virus from close contact with his son.

I was a new mom who was breast feeding. This was way before Peace management, so you can probably imagine my fear. I refused to get tested for HIV, because without a cure on the horizon, I didn't want to know the results. I couldn't allow myself to think of the possible consequences and impact on my life. I remained an ostrich with my head in the sand. Not a healthy coping mechanism, but it was all I could handle at the time. I remained in intense fear for years, until I was single again and went through HIV testing. After that episode, I told myself that I would never do mouth-to-mouth on another person again, unless it was a child.

Well again, as fate would have it, last month I went to a seminar on the effects of stress on the immune system. I was in a room with approximately 1000 people. During the seminar, someone from the back yelled "we need help back here." There was a man slumped over. At first I didn't move because I thought it was a room full of physicians and nurses. No one responded. I later found out that most of the seminar participants were psychologists and social workers. The physician presenting at the seminar was not an acute care practitioner. He went to the back of the room, but I could tell he had little exposure with arrest situations.

I headed back there, announced that I was a critical care nurse and asked if anyone else could help. Initially, no one answered. So I said "Okay then, I'm in charge until I hear differently." I quickly assessed the patient. He was not breathing. The physician was checking for a pulse. There was no pulse initially. I asked if anyone knew this man. Unfortunately, no one did. If there would have been a friend present, I would have been able to talk them through mouth-to-mouth breathing.

Well there I was, faced with a situation I had once promised myself I would never enter again, because of the years of fear I had endured. Well, I broke my promise. There, literally on my lap, on my bent knees, was a human being's head, and he was not breathing. His life was in my hands. Without another thought, I began mouth-to-mouth resuscitation. Because I am a different person than I was ten years ago, my essence has changed. I experience Peace and lack fear in general. I honestly have not experienced one ounce of fear in relation to this situation. I have not given it another thought, except telling this story to my family and now to you.

My thoughts reflect who I am. I am not a fearful person, therefore I am not spiraling down. So for me, this is a happy ending. And yes, it is an ending, I am done thinking about it. It is also a happy ending for that man who clinically died and was resuscitated. He was monitored and treated at the hospital overnight, and discharged the next day!

Hopefully, I have made it clear enough in other exercises that the fear you experience when you are faced with something that threatens your physical well being or survival is not the fear I am talking about here. That type of fear serves you well in protecting your immediate health and well-being. It is the purpose of the "fight or flight" response. The risk-benefit scale tips in your favor when the stress response kicks in during these moments. The damage that the short term stress response does on your body is far outweighed by the benefit you receive by attacking or fleeing from impending danger.

Without even realizing it, if you are to this point in the book, you may have already experienced a decrease in your fear thoughts. If so, you are on your way up the spiral.

Exercise (CC):

Eliminate the Fear

Goals for this section:

- Realize that a fearful essence is changed by having Peace in the present
- Experience Peace as a way to abolish fear

Activity:

Reflect on your improvement in the area of fear as you moved through the Peace management process. Become cognizant that you are on your way to experiencing life in a way that lacks the detrimental form of fear.

Technique: Create a New Language

This strategy was born during a moment when I was at a loss for words, and it has since taken on a life of its own.

I had spent about a half hour struggling and wrestling with my vacuum cleaner. I was unable to get the bag area released without breaking it. I was laughing at myself, saying "you are smarter than this vacuum cleaner, yet it is winning." I didn't want to bother my husband, who was involved in a project down at our barn, yet I was at a point where I was stumped. As I was walking to my cell phone to call my husband, I didn't know what I was going to say. I couldn't say that I was mad or angry. That was not what I was feeling. From the start of the wrestling match with the vacuum cleaner, I had been aware that I needed to be the gatekeeper of my Peace. If I wasn't, I could fall victim to negative emotions. From the very start, I chose Peace.

I didn't know how to communicate my need to my husband. He is one of those "knights in shining armor" types who comes to my "rescue" any time I am in need. So, if he was in the middle of something important, I didn't want him to stop. But, I needed to let him know I needed him. However, if I didn't let him know the extent of the struggle, he might wait until much later, and I really wanted him to fix the vacuum cleaner *now*. The urgency of my need was only the beginning of my dilemma. The particular choice of words actually was more confusing for me. What came out of my mouth when my husband answered the phone was something that sounded very strange to me. I said "I am dealing with a frustrating set of circumstances, and I need your help". That is not typical of my pattern of speech.

When I hung up the phone, I laughed, but I soon realized why I had said those specific, strange-sounding words. I must have innately realized that the self-fulfilling prophecy could kick into effect if I chose the wrong words.

If we say we are feeling a certain way or use emotionally descriptive words, we could subconsciously take on the energy of those emotions. The problem is that our language typically is spoken to summarize things briefly. One emotionally descriptive word communicates a great deal to the other person. But if that "emotion word" (like "angry", "mad", "frustrated", "scared") does not adequately describe what is going on inside us, we have to use several words to communicate the idea. That is why I sounded so wordy when I called my husband.

Since that day, I have observed everyone around me and their sometimes careless use of "emotion words." On occasion, the emotion word *does* seem to reflect what is going on inside of them. It is evident in their outward manifestations. This is the person in immediate need of Peace management. However, most often, I hear people using words that seem much stronger than I believe they are actually experiencing, yet their language encourages them to feel the emotion and draw out the length of the low-level charge.

I have also observed the overuse of the word "hate." I don't believe there is a word that evokes stronger negative emotion. Even before the concept of Peace management was a part of my life, I would not allow my son, or other little children I watched to use that word. I used to tell them "hate is a very ugly word". I would help them identify other words to use to describe what they felt.

This whole process of creating a new language has been a tedious, yet creative experience. Trying to find the proper words when you are communicating, while not sounding like you are from some other planet or in an ivory tower, has been a challenge. At times, I will use the old words, just because it is easier, knowing inside that they do not convey the real situation. At other times, I do carefully choose my words. At some point, down the road, our language may accurately reflect what we feel. New words may be created, or we may get used to hearing things said in a wordier manner. But for now, the accompanying exercise will simply allow you to distinguish your accurate use of "emotion words" from your exaggerations of your emotions through your choice of words.

The trick to this new language is either describing the situation or your approach rather than labeling your reaction with an "emotion word".

Rather than saying

"I am scared to drive on snow-covered roads."

say

"When the roads are snow-covered, I exercise extra caution."

This above example is perfect for observing what happens inside of you. When I say the first set of words while driving on snow covered roads, I can almost feel the fear. I find myself clutching the steering wheel tightly. When I use the second set of words, I relax into it, still remaining as cautious as I was with the first set of words, possibly even more so. There is definitely no charge while saying the second set of words.

Another strategy is to use a word that represents the negativity as outside of yourself. Therefore, it is accurate because it does not imply that you are taking on the negative emotion.

Some examples are:

instead of saying "That meeting stressed me."
say "That was a stressful meeting."

instead of saying "You made me mad."
say "You said some things that I find inconsiderate."

instead of saying "I am so worried about the results of that test."
say "Those test results will provide a lot of information."

Words are very powerful. They create much more than we would like to believe. We need to be meticulous in our thoughts and words, as they create who we are. I feel so strongly about this that I also use it in my teaching. When students are talking to patients, I encourage them to use positive phrases.

- I discourage students from saying “this medication will prevent you from rejecting your liver” to a new liver transplant patient. I ask them to say “this medication will help your body accept your new liver.”

- I discourage students from saying “this will prevent vomiting.” I ask them to say “this will make your stomach feel more settled”

You will now have an opportunity to look at your own language and use of “emotion words.”

Exercise Assignment (DD):

Create A New Language

Goals for this section:

- Raise your awareness of the frequency with which you use "emotion words"
- Identify when the "emotion words" accurately reflect your emotion
- Identify when the "emotion words" exaggerate your emotion
- Identify when the "emotion words" are used inappropriately and do not reflect an emotion but rather a situation
- Creatively develop new words to describe a formerly negatively charged situation

---

Activity A:

Attempt to monitor yourself for the frequency with which you use "emotion words." Make a mental note of your use of the following words:

angry
stressed
mad
afraid
worried
embarrassed

Do you use any other emotionally descriptive words? Do not try to correct yourself as the words are leaving your mouth, simply make a mental note. Later, when your are alone, you will engage in the activities of Exercises B and C

Activity B:

When you are alone, recall the use of the words you used above. Consider whether they accurately described your emotion or exaggerated the feeling.

Attempt to determine if by using the words, you magnified the amount of charge during the moment or prolonged the low-level charge. How long did you feel the response in your body? Did it seem more intense than it should have?

Activity C:

Try to rewrite your script during the previous conversations where you used the "emotion words."
In rewriting your script, use either the **technique of describing the situation rather than using an emotion word**

or

use the strategy of externalizing the negativity.

Here are the examples of the former strategy:

> instead of saying "I am scared to drive on snow-covered roads."
> Say "When the roads are snow-covered, I exercise extra caution."
>
> instead of saying "You made me mad."
> Say "you said some things that I find inconsiderate."

Here is an example of the latter strategy:

> instead of saying "That meeting stressed me."
> Say "That was a stressful meeting."
>
> instead of saying "I am so worried about the results of that test."
> Say "those test results will provide a lot of information."

Have fun with this one!

Technique: Peace from Total Integrity

This technique encourages you to be your *authentic self* at *ALL* times. And only *you* know if this is always occurring or not. The concept of being your authentic self means having total integrity: congruence between your desires, what you think, what you say, and what you do.

Begin by asking yourself how you would describe a person whom you feel has integrity? You might give answers like "honest," "noble," or "trustworthy." Now, describe a person whom you feel lacks integrity. Your description will most likely be opposite of the words you used above. There is obviously some difference between these individuals. Our work will be twofold. First, we must look at what creates the difference. Second, we need to realize that there is a Peace that you experience when you come from integrity. Also there is a Peace that others feel when they interact with someone who comes from a place of integrity.

Sometimes, for very strange reasons, we either deny thoughts we are having, say things we don't really mean, or act in a way that does not reflect our desires or thoughts. Maybe it is because we think these words or actions are what other people want to hear or see. Or maybe we think we will minimize conflict. Or maybe we don't want to deal with needing to change, because our complete honesty and integrity might ruffle some feathers and possibly take our life in new directions.

Whatever the reason, lack of congruency will be felt as a lack of Peace by you and will be perceived by others as a lack of honesty. Other people will pick up a subtle sadness, resentment, or agitation. These messages and behaviors will lead other people to interpret this manifested lack of congruency as dishonest.

Another very important point is that the outcome of any situation will not be your soul's desire, if your participation was based on a lack of authenticity. You cannot create situations that will allow you Peace and happiness if you are not willing to be completely honest with yourself.

One incident made this point very clear to me and my friend. Barb was dating a man we'll call Bob who lived five hours away, in Canada. I was convinced that Barb loved Bob very much and that her feelings went far beyond lust, infatuation, or superficial desires. She and Bob had endured much together. They had mature relationship skills. Yet Barb felt their relationship had hit a turning point before Easter. She was to spend Easter with Bob and his two teenage boys. She told him that she thought it would be best if they did not spend Easter together.

Barb called me, and I could hear the sadness in her heart. She said that as a result of her decision to stay home for Easter, she knew their relationship was sure to end. I asked her if she wanted it to end. She said "no." I asked her why she had decided not to go to Canada. She said, "I think Bob needs time to be alone."

I asked Barb if she had communicated what she wanted to Bob. She said "No.". I asked her what she wanted now. She said, "I want the tightest hug of my life and to cry while Bob holds me." I encouraged Barb to tell Bob that. Well, the happy ending is she called him and told him of her desire. She drove the five hours, got a huge hug, and cried in his arms.

Barb and Bob's relationship did take a turn before Easter, but it was actually a good one. They have made tremendous strides in the honesty in their communication by always striving to have congruency between their desires, thoughts, words, and actions. There is no place for repression, phoniness, or acting. There is a true freedom and Peace that comes from having integrity and being your authentic self.

You must be ruthlessly selfish and communicate your desires. You must do what is right for you, communicate it clearly, then allow the other people to do what is right for them. If you base any relationship on false information, you are not being fair to the other person either. They may be making decisions about their life based on inaccurate information. You need to be authentic and allow them the freedom to be authentic. When my authentic self meets your authentic self, we both feel greater Peace.

On the surface, others may seem like they do not want to hear what you have to say when you are being honest. It may be challenging for them. But given a few moments and some soul searching, I can't believe anyone would want you to withhold the truth that may affect them. Honesty is a risk, but one usually well worth any relatively minor stumbling blocks. I had a boyfriend who would always say "I would rather you run me down with a Mack Truck than put one brick in the road. That one brick will soon become a whole wall." What that statement did was allow me always to be open and honest with him. And in the process, I never wanted to run him down with a Mack Truck. I valued this philosophy and his spirit too much to take advantage of the situation. It made me want to nurture him and this ability and freedom.

There will be some work involved in initially getting in touch with and becoming comfortable in living out your honest desires. There is a good chance there are areas of your life where you have not been totally honest with yourself, leading to a lack of integrity.

Think back to the section "Personality Self Analysis," Are any of your labels or self descriptions blocking your ability to achieve total integrity and achieve a feeling of being your authentic self? Do you really have the freedom to be the real you? You may find it helpful to re-read that section in light of this discussion on total integrity.

The only thing standing between me (the way I am now)
and
the way I want to become
are my thoughts, words, and actions, and I control those!

To other people, the most obvious lack of congruence comes from a discrepancy between your words and your actions. When it comes to a discrepancy between your thoughts and desires with your words or actions, your acting abilities may mask some of it. If someone's words didn't match their actions, you would not trust them. This reminds me of a saying I heard long ago:

Your actions speak so loudly, I can hardly hear what you are saying.

I truly feel that if everyone, at all times, spoke and acted with integrity, there would be no room for meanness, anger, or any Peace-lacking activity. Your desire is Peace. Therefore your thoughts, words, and actions, when in congruence, would only be Peace. A lack of congruence in any one of the four components would be felt as a lack of Peace.

Having congruence means being your *authentic self.* Being your authentic self at all times will bring you the feeling of a deep sense of Peace. This is the concept I would like to leave with you.

Exercise (EE):

Peace from Total Integrity

Goals for this section:

- Explore your desires in relation to all your major life situations
- Analyze your thoughts, words, and actions, and determine if they are congruent with your desires
- Practice watching your thoughts, choosing your words and actions, and making sure they are representative of your desires

---

Activity A:

Write down your deepest desires about your major life situations. How would you like your relationship to be with a spouse or significant other? How would you like your relationship with your children to be? What are your desires about your work situation? What about any other major life situation?

Take some time to explore your desires about the following:

- friendships
- accomplishments
- home
- leisure time

- community involvement
- finances
- legacy
- free time

Activity B:

Over the course of the next several days, watch your thoughts, words, and actions. Determine if they match your soul's desire.

If they do not, analyze what is blocking your honesty and creating the lack of congruence.

What happens in your body when you are not experiencing a congruence between your desires and your thoughts, actions, or words? Use this feeling to begin guiding your future expression of your desires. The same feelings will come up for you, in relation to big or small desires.

Make a commitment to constantly monitor the congruence between your desires and your thoughts, words, and actions.

Are you aware of Peace when you are your authentic self?

Part 4:

Forming A Group

9 Suggestions for a Group & the Facilitator

My hope is that people who learn Peace management will share it and support others on their personal quest for Peace. This can be done one-on-one with a spouse, child, parent, friend, or co-worker, and it can also be done through a support group or study group.

I have specified both "support group" and "study group" because they take on slightly different purposes. Both groups involve study and support, but the emphasis is slightly different.

A *study group* will take the book, section by section, analyze it, determine plans for applying suggestions, discuss the concepts in detail, then report back to the group with the success or obstacles found in applying the concepts. The group often helps the individuals with applying the concepts successfully. Usually, in the process, the group also serves as a support system for each member.

A *support group* focuses more on the discussion of how each person is progressing, in this case with becoming a better Peace manager. The group realizes that it is not an easy task and develops ideas and strategies to help each individual. In the process, you may study and discuss concepts that are outlined in the book.

In the initial stage of the group discussions, you should determine which type of group you are, to eliminate any confusion or frustration members may have about the purpose and focus of the group. This will help members know what they can expect from the group.

Both types of groups work well with Peace management. If you decide to work through the book as a group program, it should take around 15 - 20 weeks to get through the whole book. However, the pace is really determined by the group.

My suggestion is that, once the purpose and flow of the group is established, you do not change it unless it is *really* not working well. If you sense the group plan is not working well, bring your concern to the attention of the group. Changes should be made only when agreed upon by the group. Once, I was in what I believed was a very effective and stimulating study group. The facilitator acted on some things she did not understand (most of us engaged in purposeful conversations that were a spin off of the readings at hand) She just announced immediate changes that were to be implemented without any discussion or input from the other members. She thought she was doing a good job as the facilitator. What she did not take into account is that several of the group members had been in study groups together in the past. This group fell into a pattern that worked for them without ever discussing the format as a group.

In that moment, the whole "feel" of the group changed. We tried it her way, however the conversation felt very stifled and it did not allow the members the free-flow feeling of applying the information from other creative works that we enjoyed. Up to that point, the discussions had been very lively and stimulating and I sensed tremendous growth in all of us. By simply sticking to the readings at hand, I came away feeling "I can read the book on my own. Growth comes from exploring the concept with other like-minded individuals."

At the end of the meeting, I asked the group if it was going to continue in the new format. Everyone just shrugged and basically answered "I guess". At that point, I stated that I knew this new format would not meet my needs and I would bow out of the group. I asked them to let me know if they ever decided to go back to the old format. I soon found another group that was in synch with my goals. The group I left had been meeting weekly for several months, but within one month, the group dissolved.

The lesson is: be clear in the beginning about the purpose, focus, and intention of the group and then don't make any changes unless it is decided by the group, as a whole.

As a facilitator, you can decide if the group will be a study group or support group, and then publicize it that way. Or you can just say you would like to have a discussion group about Peace management, and the group can determine the purpose at your first meeting.

Groups can be started with neighbors or friends, however, a small advertisement in a local publication may add to its numbers. I must say you get a more diversified group when you advertise in a newspaper, and diversity enriches the group.

These meetings could be held in someone's home, at a local bookstore or library, community center, or church. Usually, there is a nominal charge for the use of these types of facilities for meetings. Remember, convenience is definitely a bonus. However, people will often make extraordinary efforts to attend groups they find effective and stimulating.

Meetings should have a time limit, and one person should be asked to watch the clock. My suggestion is about 90 minutes. Shorter than that time frame doesn't allow the group to get deep into discussion. If meetings are longer than that, people may begin to feel as though the group is infringing on too much of their time.

If you feel the discussion is really getting to the meat of an issue when you run out of time, you may want to take the meeting elsewhere (another room or to a local coffee house). This way, no one feels obligated to stay past the 90 minutes or feel like they are abandoning their group. I do not suggest lengthening the meeting because you might be setting a pattern that some might not find acceptable. Some members may feel they will burn out on the topic if meetings are too long.

Offering beverages is fine, however, I do not suggest providing food at group meetings, because it changes the meeting to feel like a social gathering. Also, if food is provided, people might feel an obligation to take turns providing food and their finances or time schedule might not permit this. The sense of obligation might be enough to make them feel uncomfortable and bow out of the group.

I suggest finding a place that has minimal distractions. If you meet in a home, don't meet where someone has small children or a spouse who watches the TV with the volume up high. If you decide to meet in a public place, go check it out for distractions and other events that may cause a conflict with your meetings.

It should also be decided whether newcomers will be allowed to join the group once the group begins. Keeping an open-door policy has been common practice in most of the groups I have joined. The meetings have been very free-flowing. Whoever shows up that night is part of the discussion. I have not found this fluidity to be difficult. The new person is briefly caught up and jumps right in. But the decision to allow new members should be a group decision, because it might change the dynamics of the group.

The facilitator will also want to consider the number in the group. I have been in groups made up of only 3 core individuals who worked very well together and in much larger groups. Just be aware that if there are many more than 10 in a group, each person will not have as much time to speak or ask questions.

I suggest that the group determines some ground rules during the first meeting. I always have my nursing students do this when they are in my class participating in Peace management groups. I have asked them to write down their rules so I could share them in this book as a way to provide ideas. Here are some of my students' suggestions:

- What is discussed in the group stays in the group. This really builds a sense of trust and provides a safe feeling to be open with thoughts and feelings.
- Don't interrupt when someone else is talking.
- If you disagree with someone, be respectful in your approach.
- Try not to dominate the conversation, unless you are having a particularly difficult time with something.
- When helping a member of the group, everyone should make suggestions rather then tell the person what to do.
- If you do not want to be part of the discussion on any particular topic, let the group know.
- Everyone is allowed equal talk time.

The group is yours, so do as you like. However, you may want to give some thought as to the format of the meeting. You may choose a format where the facilitator determines what section of the book will be discussed at the next meeting. Each participant comes to the meeting having read the section and ready to discuss. Or you may choose to read a section together at the meeting, discussing as you go along or at the end of the section.

You can also determine if the group will be more free-flowing or if the facilitator will go around the room asking for input from each person. If you choose the second option, you may want to adopt some way that a member can let the group know if they do not choose to speak at present. You may say "pass" or "I don't have anything to add at this time." No one should be made to feel that they have to contribute on every topic.

As far as the facilitator goes, personality does not seem to matter. In my nursing student groups, I purposely pick group leaders with very different personality styles. The feedback I elicit from the students demonstrates that the personality of the leader does not matter, as long as they take the role seriously and keep the group focused.

As a facilitator, your job is to keep the conversation flowing, make sure the group is acting in accordance with the established ground rules, and handle all of the behind the scene details. Sometimes it is felt that the facilitator should have a better understanding of the concepts, or at least more experience with the topic, but that is not always feasible. You might want to read the information to be discussed at the meeting ahead of time though, to have a general list of questions you may want to pose to the group.

I would like to bring something else to your attention. The work of Peace management does not occur in the group sessions. Although conflicts may arise, which would require you to practice Peace during a group session, the sessions are not where the work is done. The work is done in the other six days, twenty two and a half hours. You practice Peace management when you are confronted with choices, experiencing moments, serving in your roles, and standing in the middle of chaos.

The group simply serves as the forum for you to discuss concepts and your efforts to apply them. Peace is actually a passive state, but the process of moving toward it is work. In the beginning, Peace management will be a process. Eventually it will be a way of "being."

Having participated in many and varied study and support groups, I am a strong advocate for this type of learning. I process information more quickly and find creative ways to apply information. I also utilize the groups as a sounding board for my interpretation of concepts. Whether you choose a study group or support group, you are likely to find a group helpful to your process of developing into a skilled Peace manager.

Part 5:

Pathophysiology of Stress

10 AGAIN, THE NEED FOR PEACE MANAGEMENT

co-authored by James Landis, M.D., Ph.D., CSCS

Your body is an awesome piece of machinery. It is a finely tuned, adaptive organism. The top engineers from the best universities couldn't design such a marvel. There are a number of chemicals circulating in your blood at any given time. There are a number of areas that manufacture and store these chemicals, and you have a number of cells and tissues that respond to these chemicals in a very typical and predictable way. One, specific version of this process occurs as your body responds to stress.

Occasionally, this stress-response design is helpful. The intention of these chemicals, and the cascade of occurrences related to the chemicals, was intended to preserve your existence. However, at times these chemicals are harmful to us. The focus of this chapter is the effect of the chemicals released during unwarranted, perceived stress, anger, and other emotions that carry a charge. When the body's stress response is triggered during an unnecessary perception of immediate stress or in a habitual unwarranted way, our health is compromised.

The design of the stress response is to assure us that we have all the resources we need at a time of extreme stress. That is the "fight or flight" response mentioned in the beginning of the book. The benefit of the fight or flight response is that it can save your life when you are in danger of falling victim to a potentially harmful or fatal event, such as encountering an angry tiger.

I don't think many of you will be dealing with tigers that could maim or kill you, unless you are performers in Las Vegas (sorry, guys!). Our bodies, however, do not register the difference between truly threatening situations and mundane circumstances in which we experience stress. The body's response to stress, which includes the entangled workings of the nervous system, (the brain and the peripheral nerves), the endocrine system, (the glands and hormones), the blood, and immune system, can actually create dysfunction and disease.

Over the past 30 years, a whole field of study has developed to address this phenomenon. Psychoneuroimmunology, or PNI, studies the way diseases are caused by our emotions and thoughts. We also have a new vocabulary word in health care: *allostatic load.* The term allostatic refers to cumulative negative effects or the *wear and tear* placed on the body relative to stress.

Hang with us. You decided to read this. Remember it was optional. If you are having second thoughts, here is your chance to bow out gracefully.

Remember, the whole process starts with a thought. You have a thought that *you perceived* as stressful:

- "The wind is blowing very hard and the cracking sound I just heard is that huge tree limb falling in my direction."
- "Oh, there is my father. He is probably going to tell me how I messed up my life again."
- "How am I going to get this all done before my boss gets back in town?"

You have carte blanche approval from us to "turn on" the stress response system if that huge tree limb is falling your way (or in any similar such life threatening situation). However, you potentially damage your health if you activate your stress response in situations similar to the last two situations. Why? The simple answer is your life is not in danger in those type of situations. Ironically, you are creating a dangerous situation where none exists. As a result, the true danger is from within rather than from something external. The chemicals released in your body, due to your perception and activation of the stress response, becomes dangerous if you repeatedly turn on the stress response in a very non-necessary, habitual pattern.

Note that above we chose to use the words *you perceived.* That is because, when it comes to psychological stress, it is all about perception. It is your thoughts and the meaning that you give to them. If your back was turned and you did not see your father enter the room, would you still feel stressed? Probably not. However, when you saw him, you created a thought that ultimately triggered the stress response.

The thought probably arose in the part of your brain called the cerebral cortex. The cortex is that outside layer of the brain, sometimes referred to as the gray matter, though other important areas of gray matter exist in the central nervous system. In illustrations, the cerebral cortex is the part of the brain that looks convoluted (lumpy), or like a pile of large, cooked macaroni. Essentially, your brain is made up nerve cell tissue and structural tissue. The nerve cells communicate with other portions of your brain in bi-directional (two-way) and multidirectional ways and often, communicate with different portions of your body.

The *limbic system* of the brain is sometimes called the emotional center of the brain. There are several structures which are in close proximity in the middle of your brain that make up this system. This is the system that you utilize to identify some event or occurrence as stressful, and in turn, it activates the response which we usually refer to as the emotion. Ultimately, the limbic system seems to help link the thought with the body response, which we call the feeling.

As previously stated in the main text of this book, you cannot control what happens after you have the thought. It is an automatic response. The resulting process is controlled by two systems:

- the Autonomic Nervous System
- your neuroendocrine system, which is a combined system of your nervous system and your endocrine system. The nervous system includes the brain, spinal cord, and nerves. The endocrine system includes glands and the hormones that they secrete.

You must control the thought or the ***meaning you give to the thought*** *in an effort not to trigger the stress response.* THIS IS THE WHOLE CRUX OF PEACE MANAGEMENT.

Well let's pretend you jumped ahead to this section of the book and you are not a skilled Peace manager yet. What happens after you have a thought that you perceive as stressful? There are two major systems that are activated simultaneously.

The first system activated (see figure 1) is the one that is manifested in a very rapid manner. It is the Autonomic Nervous System (ANS). The ANS has two distinct, and often opposing branches. Those two branches are the Sympathetic Nervous System and the Parasympathetic Nervous System. Both systems get their information from either the brain or from various organs in the body. For our purpose, we are concerned with the information the ANS receives from the brain, as the brain is where stress is perceived.

The stressful information activates the Sympathetic branch of the ANS. Information acknowledging stress travels to the Hypothalamus of the brain, then to the brain stem. The response to this information subsequently leaves the central nervous system (the brain and spinal cord) and travels though the peripheral nervous system (the nerves out in the body). This response/information is

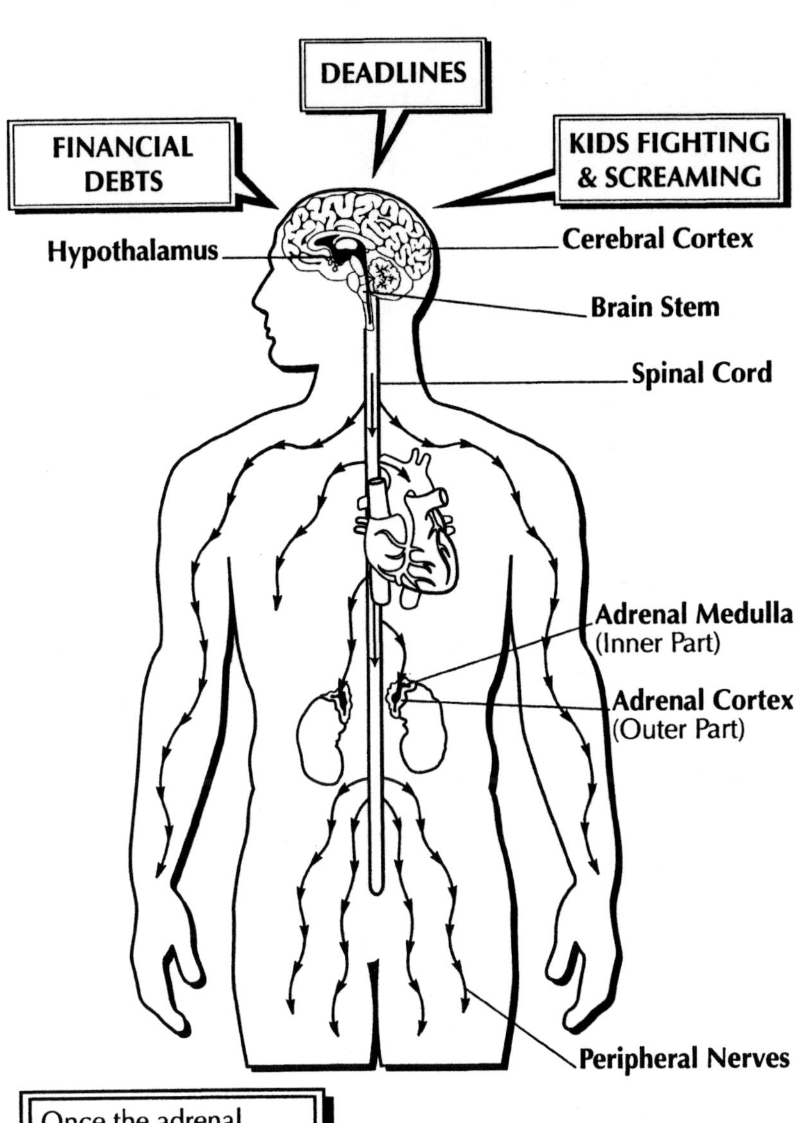

Once the adrenal medulla is stimulated directly by the nerve, it releases epinephrine & norepinephrine directly into the blood.

ACTIVATION OF THE AUTONOMIC NERVOUS SYSTEM

FIGURE 1

communicated via an electrochemical system. Neurons (nerve cells) form a path to an end organ or a blood vessel. Neurons in the body (similar to neurons in the brain) have a very specific way of communicating.

A neuron (see figure 2) has receiving parts, called dendrites. They converge on the nerve cell body. The impulse-exit portion of the nerve cell is an extension called the axon. In the end of the axon, neurotransmitters (chemical messengers) are synthesized and then stored in tiny vesicles (bubbles), awaiting a specific signal to be released. The electrical information (a change in negative/positive charge, where the inside of the cell becomes more positive, thus "depolarizing" the membrane) travels from the dendrite to the cell body and finally to the axon. Upon reaching the end of the axon, the current of electricity cues a sequence of events, ultimately causing the vesicles to release the neurotransmitter chemicals into the synapse (space between nerve cells or between nerve cell and a gland or muscle).

There are two neurotransmitters utilized by the nerves in the Sympathetic Nervous System. The most important neurotransmitter, which directly influences the tissues of your body to act a certain way is called norepinephrine. Norepinephrine binds to a structure on the membrane of a cell called a receptor. Thus, when the neurotransmitter binds to the cell membrane receptor, it can either excite or inhibit particular actions of that cell. It can cause its effect in one of two ways. It can either change the permeability (permissiveness of substances to enter the next cell), allowing electrically charged ions to enter the cell, or it can act directly on the cell. An example of these types of actions would be allowing calcium to enter the cell. Should the cell happen to be a part of the smooth muscle of a blood vessel, the calcium would enable the muscle to contract. If this scenario were to occur often enough, one can easily envision blood vessel constriction or narrowing, and increased blood pressure as a result.

This may all seem very complex, but the ANS functions in such a well-defined and finely tuned way and responds appropriately

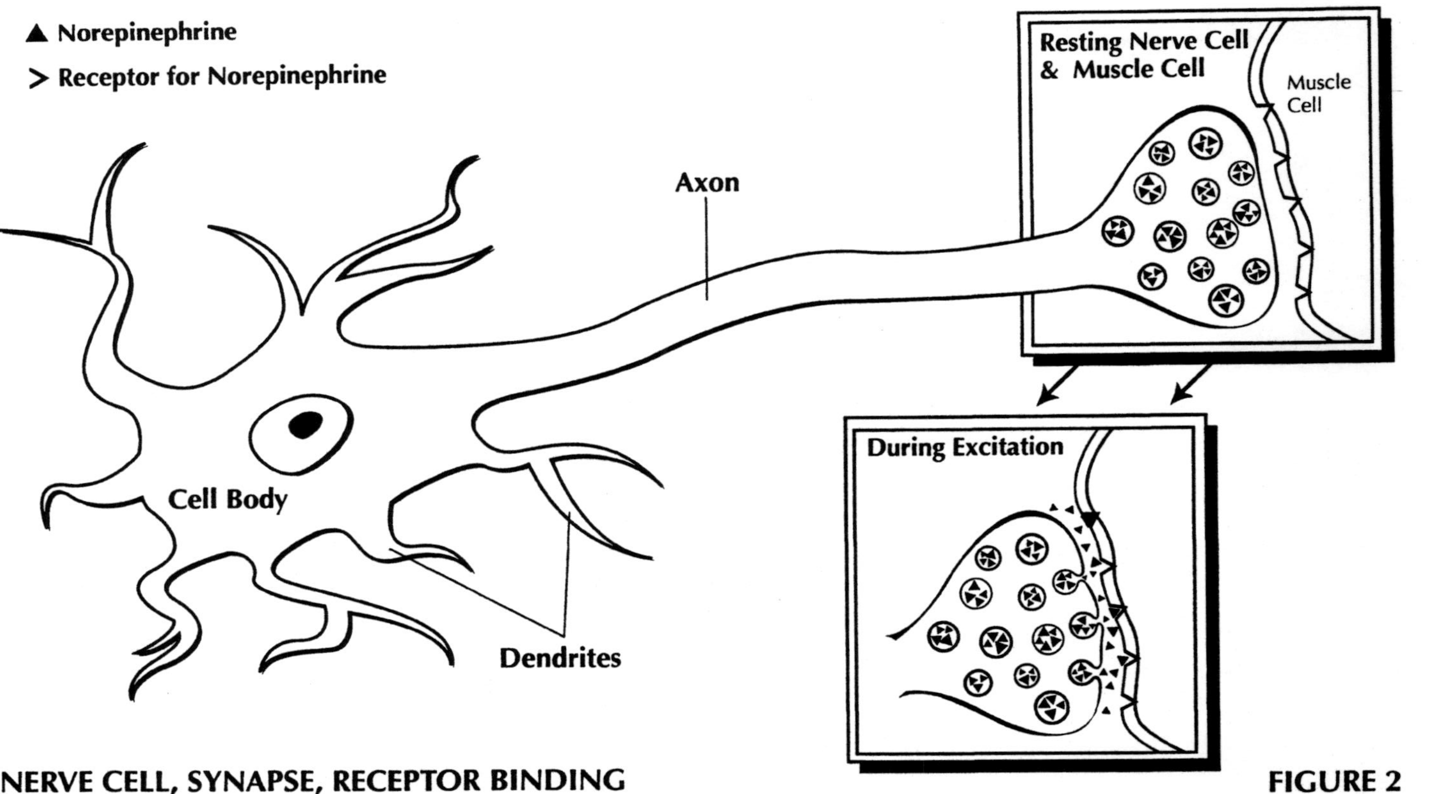

NERVE CELL, SYNAPSE, RECEPTOR BINDING

FIGURE 2

within milliseconds. It can cause very substantial effects in a very short period of time. In fact, it has been previously demonstrated that "within 3 to 5 seconds [the ANS] can increase the heart rate to twice normal, and within 10 to 15 seconds the arterial blood pressure can be doubled" (Guyton and Hall, 697). The systemic arterial blood pressure is commonly referred to as simply your blood pressure, typically averaging 120/80 ("120 over 80"). Are you beginning to see the dangers of having a stress response when it is not really needed to preserve your life? Just imagine what a doubled blood pressure would do to a weakened blood vessel (an aneurysm) or how hard a weak heart would have to work to pump blood out into a system with such a high pressure.

Just as a side note, the Sympathetic Nervous System (SNS) and Parasympathetic Nervous System (PSNS) are never turned off. They are never asleep. They are just in low gear, keeping a fine balance. In fact, the Sympathetic Nervous System normally keeps the blood vessels in the body about 50% constricted (tightened). The blood vessels are never totally relaxed, except in rare circumstances (like in a quadriplegic patient who loses control of the autonomic nerves or after prolonged frostbite where there is a paralysis of blood vessels).

The second important function of the SNS is release/secretion of the adrenal medulla's hormones (which also serve as neurotransmitters). The adrenal glands are small glands that sit on top of each kidney. Functionally, there are two parts of the adrenal gland. The outer part is called the cortex and the inner portion is called the medulla.

When the SNS is activated, there is a direct nerve path into the medulla of the adrenal gland. This causes the adrenal medulla to secrete epinephrine, also known as adrenaline, and to a much lesser extent norepinephrine. Both chemicals are called catecholamines and are secreted directly into the bloodstream. The catecholamines travel to every organ in your body. Their effect is as intense as the nerve cell release of norepinephrine. However, though the response is slower to initiate, their effect is much longer lasting. Guyton & Hall state that the effects of the circulating catecholamines last 5 to 10 times as long as the effects that are a *direct stimulation* by the ANS (703).

There are many tissues influenced by these catecholamines, but the cardiovascular system is arguably the most profoundly affected. Epinephrine makes the heart beat much faster and stronger, and norepinephrine predominately constricts the blood vessels. They are very potent chemicals and have very dramatic effects. These catecholamines are so powerful that these are actually the type of chemicals we give in medication form to patients who are in shock (potentially fatal low blood pressure). These two chemicals have a great deal of similarity; in fact epinephrine is a precursor (forming substance for) norepinephrine. These chemicals bind to what are called adrenergic receptors throughout the body. They are the predominant chemicals associated with the fight or flight response.

The SNS gets the body ready immediately to act in a necessary, self-preserving way, should you be faced with a life threatening situation. It gets you primed to handle the situation appropriately. Unfortunately, these same chemicals are released when your wife threatens to divorce you.

Simultaneous with the activation of the SNS, your brain activates the Limbic-Hypothalamic-Pituitary-Adrenal Axis (LHPA). This system is somewhat slower to respond, but the effect lasts much longer than the effects from stimulation of the ANS. It also has been implicated in a gradual wearing down of certain parts of the body.

In this LHPA system (see figure 3), similar to activation of the ANS, the Limbic System perceives the stress. However, in this axis, when the Hypothalamus is activated it releases corticotropin-releasing hormone (CRH) into a vein that travels to the anterior lobe (front part) of the master gland of the body, the pituitary gland. Both lobes are important in controlling many functions of the body, but it is the anterior lobe, also known as the adenohypophysis, that plays a role in the stress response.

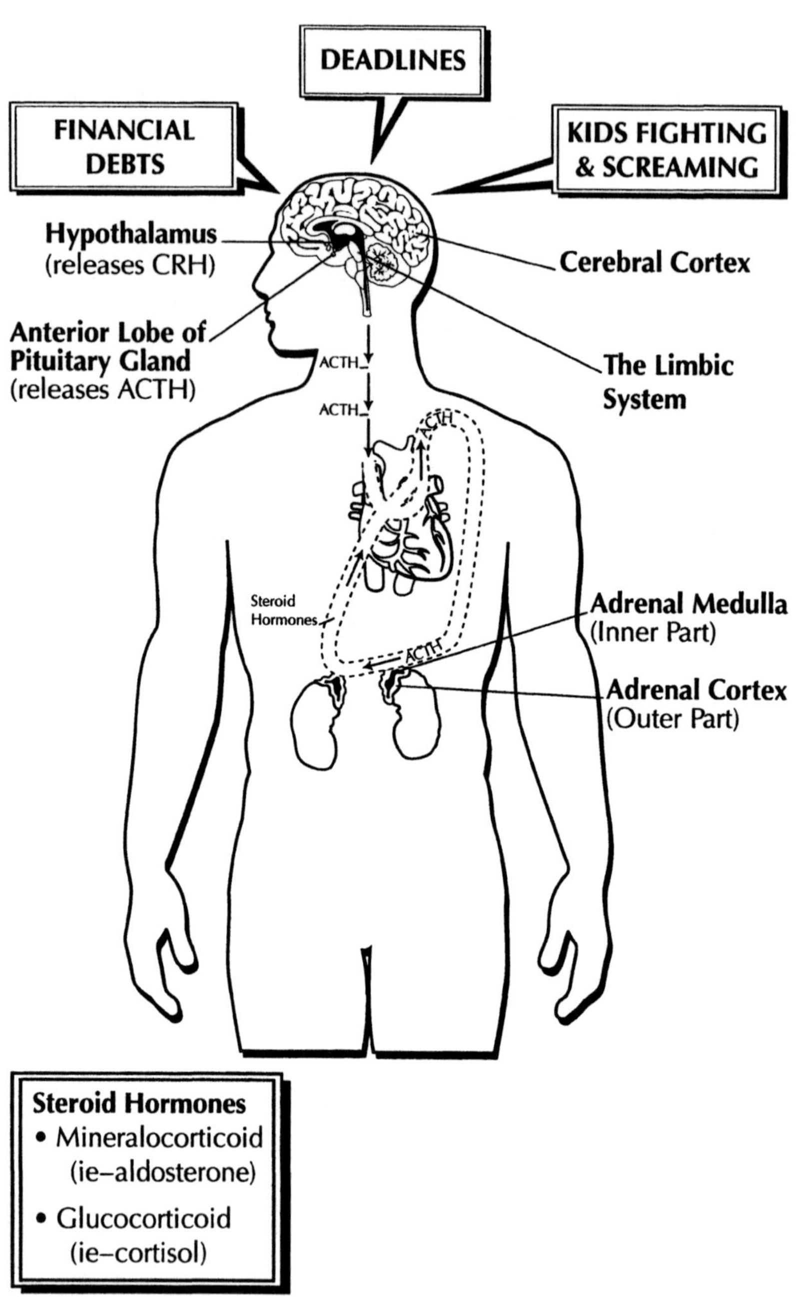

ACTIVATION OF LHPA SYSTEM
(Limbic–Hypothalamus–Pituitary–Adrenal)

FIGURE 3

The anterior lobe of the pituitary gland responds to CRH by releasing other hormones, one of which is called Adrenocorticotropic Hormone (ACTH). This hormone is released into the general circulation (the blood stream). When it reaches the outer portion of the adrenal glands, called the adrenal cortices (cortex), the glands release various steroid hormones (no, not the kind taken by some athletes and the Governor of California). There are two main categories of these steroid hormones: glucocorticoids and mineralocorticoids. The major mineralocorticoid, which accounts for 90% of all mineralocorticoid activity, is called aldosterone. The main function of aldosterone is to force the body not to urinate out as much sodium and water. This allows a larger volume of fluid to remain in the blood, which can aid in keeping the blood pressure elevated. However, it should be noted that ACTH is only a minor stimulus for the release of aldosterone. It does stimulate the release of glucocorticoids, some of which can have an effect on blood pressure much like aldosterone, especially when present in high levels, for extended periods of time.

The other category of steroid hormones, glucocorticoids, is very active in the stress response. The major glucocorticoid in humans is cortisol. Cortisol, also known as hydrocortisone, is very potent and accounts for 95% of all glucocorticoid activity. One of the main functions of cortisol is assuring there is enough glucose (usable sugar) available in the blood for the extra activity that may be needed during stressful episodes. It can provide extra glucose to the body in many ways. Three of these ways are

- making the liver convert glycogen (the stored version of glucose) to glucose
- making the body use proteins and other substances to form glucose; called gluconeogenesis
- preventing the body from converting the sugar and storing it as fat

Can you see how all these mechanisms could be very harmful to a person who has Diabetes and already has trouble lowering their blood sugar?

Although raising the blood sugar can be very harmful in some individuals, there are other effects of cortisol that are more harmful and potentially more devastating: the effects of immunosuppression (halting of the immune system) and inflammatory alterations. These are very well known effects of cortisol. In fact, in health care, we often administer medications which are synthetic and more potent versions of cortisol, namely Cortisone, Prednisone, Methylprednisone, and Dexamthasone. They are given in an effort to suppress the immune system or stop an inflammatory process. One reasonable use of these medications is in people who have received organ transplants. They suppress the immune system so that the new organ is less likely to be rejected.

Once the cortisol is released into the blood system, it triggers many cells and parts of the immune system to suppress certain cells and activate other cells. Once the levels of cortisol reach a high enough level in the blood, it starts something called a negative feedback system which down-regulates the LHPA axis. This will decrease the continued release of cortisol. This process of repeated turning-on and turning-off could interfere with the normal circadian rhythmic release of cortisol. The term "circadian" refers to the normal variation of cortisol levels throughout the day. The level of cortisol that is produced by our body to optimize bodily functions is a very fine-tuned mechanism. Therefore, the more control you exert over unnecessary psychological stress, the less likely you will be to disrupt the finely tuned circadian rhythm release of cortisol.

The effect of cortisol on the immune system is fairly widespread, affecting various components of the system. Because the immune system is probably more complex than we actually understand at this point, it is probably best to focus on certain well understood general effects. Indeed, according to Huether and McCance, cortisol acts at several sites to influence immune and inflammatory reactions. It does such things as depress proliferation of T lymphocytes, including those that produce the antiviral protein interferon; decrease natural killer cell activity; reverse macrophage activity; decrease the number of eosinophils and fibroblasts; and suppress the synthesis, secretion, and action of chemical mediators involved in inflammatory and immune responses (465).

Also, according to Robert Sapolsky, a Stanford University professor and oft-cited scientist and author, "a period of stress will disrupt a wide variety of immune functions. Stress will suppress the formation of new lymphocytes and their release into circulation, and shortens the time preexisting lymphocytes stay in circulation. It will inhibit the manufacturing of new antibodies in response to an infectious agent, and disrupt communication between lymphocytes though release of relevant messengers" (151).

So, while we might regale you with evidence and expert opinion, at this point it might be helpful to fill in a few details about the immune system. Much of the function of the immune system revolves around the function of the white blood cells (WBC), "the *mobile units* of the body's protective system." (Guyton, 392). WBCs start as something called a stem cell (see figure 4). They begin their life and development in the bone marrow and lymph tissue. From the stem cell, the WBC is designated to develop into one of several cell types. There are two major classifications of WBC: the myelocytes and lymphocytes. The myelocytes are well suited to engulfing and destroying infected or foreign cells. In their adult form, the myeloctes/monocytes are most often referred to as macrophages. However, while all white blood cells have a role in fighting infection or inflammation, and are influenced by stress, it is the lymphocytes that are the most directly and greatly affected by stress.

The first lineage of white blood cells, the myeloid lineage, has two lines for further division. The *first line* is made up of the granulocytes. The three categories of granulocytes are neutrophils, eosinophils, and basophils. The *second line* is the monocytes. After being released from their birth place, monocytes are released into the blood stream. They find a home in body tissue and mature into macrophages. Macrophages become relatively large, very powerful immune cells. One type of macrophage is called the Kupfer cells. They are the work horse for cleaning the blood in the liver. One macrophage can ingest and kill 100 bacteria cells. Compared to the

Stem Cell
Natural Killer Cell
Myeloid Lineage (myelocytes)
Lymphoid Lineage (lymphocytes)
Granulocytes
Monocytes
B Cell
T Cell
Neutrophils
Eosinophils
Basophils
Travels to Tissue
Macrophage

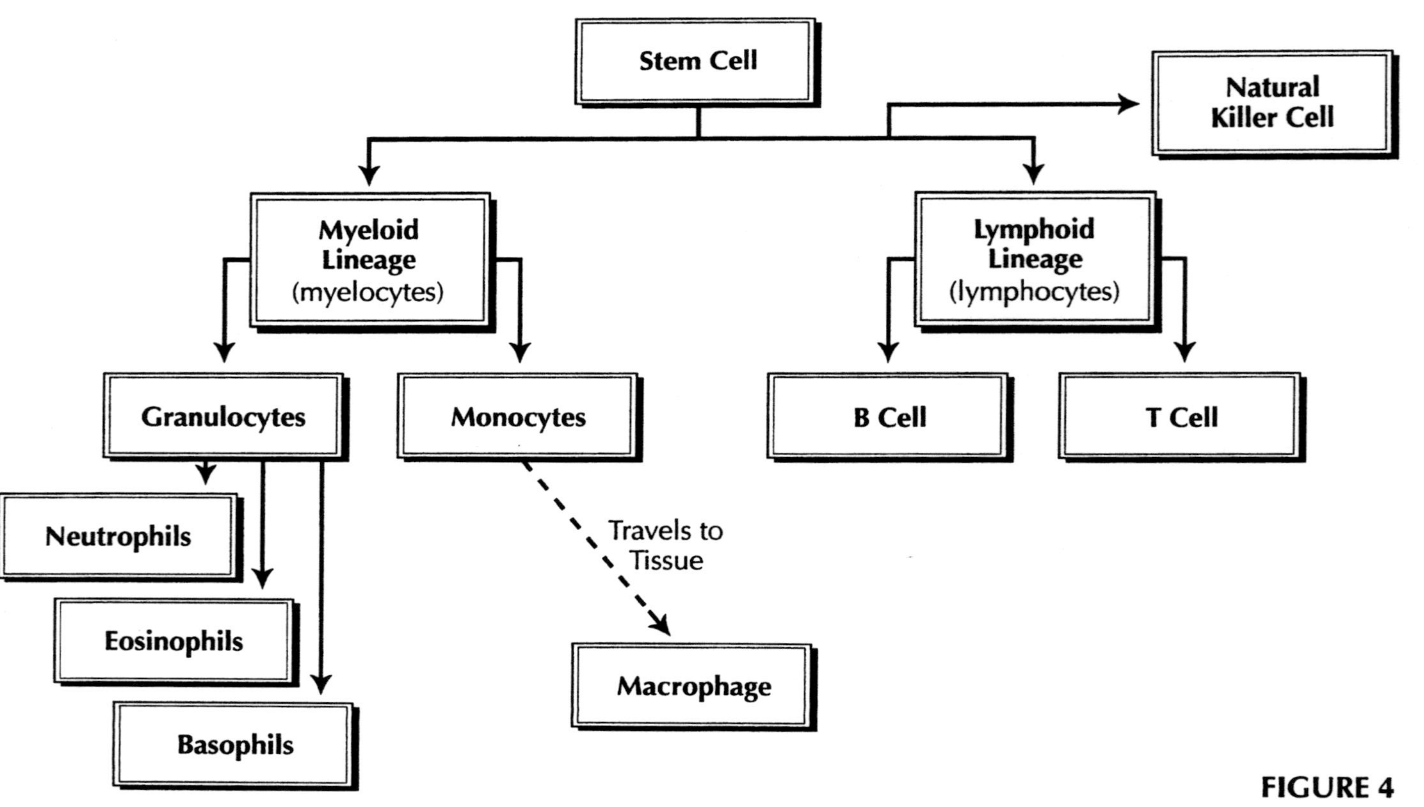

FIGURE 4

second lineage, these cells are more general killers—killing things they know do not belong to the body.

The cells of the lymphoid lineage represents a class of invader-destroyer cells, typified by the B and T cells. If the lymphoid WBC matures in the bone marrow, it will most likely become a B cell. If it matures in the thymus gland, which lies in the front of the chest, just above the heart, it will become a T cell. The B cell eventually becomes a plasma cell of the blood. As a mature plasma cell, the B cell can be called upon to manufacture antibodies. You've probably heard of antibodies. They're the proteins that are made by the B cells as a response to a specific antigen (body invader). Antibodies are generally quite specific to the antigen for which they were created. The antibodies adhere to the antigens by binding to them. Binding with the invader essentially renders it useless or targets it for disposal, so that it cannot do harm in the body.

T cells, on the other hand, do not produce antibodies. They instead mature as specifically targeted against one particular antigen. The process of T cell development continues until there are different T cells with specific reactivites against literally millions of different antigens. These different types of processed T cells leave the thymus, traveling through the blood stream, and take up residence in lymph nodes all over the body (Guyton & Hall, 403-404). Basically, each T cell becomes the immune system's quick answer to the threat of a given antigen.

There is an additional type of lymphoid cell that develops into a specific immune cell. They are called natural killer cells. They can destroy cells that are infected with viruses and some types of cancer cells. As mentioned earlier, cortisol decreases the natural killer cell activity.

Other important, but non-cellular components of the immune system that are altered by stress are known as the cytokines. Cytokines are chemical messengers that are made and released by either the monocytes or macrophages or the lymphocytes. Some of the classifications for these messengers are the interferons, the interleukins, and tumor necrosis factor. The cytokines form the primary mechanism which either wakes up, revs up, stops, or instructs the various immune cells to respond to a stressful event, or a potentially harmful invader and orchestrate the defense process.

Remember earlier when we noted that the immune system is probably more complex than we actually understand at this point? Well, that statement derives in part from the sometimes paradoxical relationship between stress and the immune response. For example, stress can also *trigger* or *suppress* the inflammatory response of the body through release of the cytokines. Stress causes the release of some proinflammatory messengers, which causes inflammation, and some anti-inflammatory messengers, which will prevent certain types of inflammation. The danger, of course, comes when stress creates or perpetuates inflammation to the point that it becomes harmful, or if it suppresses inflammation at a time when it is really needed.

Now that you know some of the basics of the immune system and its relationship with stress, it's time to push forward and tighten the message. That is to say, "How does any of this really relate to health, wellness, and disease?" Well, as you might expect, the answers are not always clear-cut and remain somewhat speculative, but there are some important clues that suggest how stress might be related to disease. For example, one of the continuing mysteries of medicine involves the potential, varied causes of autoimmune disease.

The phrase "autoimmune disease" refers to a type of disease process that is thought to be a result of an immune system that has gone awry. As you know, your immune system is designed to recognize the cells of your body that belong there (your liver cell, your blood cell, and so on) and leave them alone. This is known as *self recognition.* Alternately, the immune system is also designed to recognize things that do not belong (viruses, bacteria, cancer cells) and destroy them because they are *nonself.* An autoimmune disease results when your immune system does not recognize some appropriate part of you (*self*) and instead treats it as *nonself,* ultimately damaging or destroying those parts of you. It is a form of unintentional *internal suicide*, in which a part of your body may be literally killing itself. The specific disease that arises depends on the particular cells that are attacked.

Now, during stress, there is an imbalance in a type of immune cells. This imbalance is known as a Th2 shift. Huether and McCance explain that under certain conditions, a [Th2] shift can induce proinflammatory activities and from these mechanisms may influence the onset or course of autoimmune/inflammatory, allergic, and neoplastic (cancer) diseases, and infections (229).

Sapolsky presents an explanation of how this might occur. He suggests the possibility that numerous, transient stressors and the repeated ups and downs of cortisol release may ratchet the stress/immune system balance upward, biasing it toward autoimmunity (p. 159). The idea is that perhaps the cortisol level never has a chance to come back to baseline. Therefore, there isn't adequate recovery time between sequential stress response activations. With each step up the "stress staircase," the baseline cortisol level rests at a new set point, and it increases with each sequential stressor. Phrased differently, as your body attempts to recover to a "normal" baseline level of cortisol in your blood, another stress sends the level up again. This scenario is repeated over and over, until eventually the cortisol levels remain high enough for a long enough period of time, that the mysterious mechanisms of autoimmune disease become manifest.

More recently (Epel, et al), evidence has emerged that suggests stress may disrupt your health by affecting the very strands of DNA in your cells. This particular report noted that women with higher psychological stress levels have shorter telomeres (the ends of the DNA strands) in their circulating immune cells. Telomeres are important because they play a role in cellular aging and the overall stability of genes. They actually shorten with each round of cell replication. Thus, the older the individual, the shorter the telomeres will be. Interesting, but here's the real kicker: the difference in telomere shortening between stressed-out study participants and the "normal" control group was equal to nearly 10 years of additional aging.

These findings imply a cellular mechanism for how chronic stress may cause the onset of some diseases. Chronically, stress would appear to potentially shorten the lives of immune cells. This is compelling stuff, but future studies will need to expand to other cell types and the potential effects will need to be observed over longer periods of time.

A final warning from Gina Marie: Overall, the body of the medical literature is filled with information which suggests links between stress and the worsening of specific disease processes. However, because I have spent my entire career as a cardiac nurse, I would be remiss if I did not offer a few words of warning to any potential cardiac disease victims: please become a Peace manager!

I have long perceived a consistent correlation between stress and cardiac disease. Imagine for a moment how taxing it must be for your heart and blood vessels to be revved up on a regular basis. I'm not talking about short bouts of exercise here . . . those are good for you! Your heart is not designed to have a rapid rate all the time. Also, your coronary arteries, the vessels that feed your heart fresh oxygen and nutrients, fill up during the rest period of your heart beat. If you have a fast heart rate, you shorten the filling time of your coronary arteries. If this filling rate is consistently shortened, your heart muscle tends to be somewhat deprived of the necessary oxygen and nutrients. This deprivation of the heart muscle potentially initiates heart rhythm disturbances, which are well known to result in the heart's being an inefficient pump.

Further, stress causes you to exhibit a high blood pressure. What that means for your heart is a tougher time pumping blood out into the high pressure circulation. An easy way to demonstrate this is to put a straw in your mouth and blow out. Then, try it a second time. This time, pinch the straw half way, simulating higher pressure in the straw. Can you see how much harder you have to blow to get the air through the straw? This is the same thing that happens with your heart. It is this hard work that can change the heart muscle in ways that are ultimately very ominous for your health.

If that's not enough, well then there's always the concept that chronic high blood pressure can more easily force fats into the blood vessel wall, especially where vessels branch off into two (bifurcate). The whirling of blood (turbulence) at this bifurcation injures the lining of the blood vessel and then allows the accumulation of cholesterol-rich fat into the lining of the blood vessel wall. The proper name for this condition is "atherosclerosis," and it is as widespread in America as mobile phones and blue jeans.

This fat deposit (atherosclerotic plaque) causes a narrowing of the blood vessel. Blood slows through this narrow passageway and sluggish blood flow lends itself to blood clot formation. A vessel choked off by a clot would no longer supply blood to the area beyond the blockage. This type of blockage, of course, is what causes most heart attacks, (which are death of part of the heart muscle), and strokes. However, even without something as potentially catastrophic at tissue death, tissues and organs can become very distressed and lose appreciable function simply from the fat deposit-induced reduction of blood flow. Simply put, your organs can only handle so much malnutrition/ischemia (lack of blood supply) before they become sick or injured.

Adding it all up, a "malnourished" heart muscle can cause potentially dangerous heart rhythm disturbances, which could then lead to further interference of the blood supply to the heart muscle, which could worsen the rhythm disturbance, which could then decrease blood flow, which lived in the house that Jack built...well, you get it, right? A vicious cycle is created and maintained. Preventing an unnecessary stress response through Peace management is a way to be kind to your heart and other organs.

The conditions and diseases listed below have been cited throughout the medical literature to either be directly related to stress, exacerbated by stress, or be an indirect result of the stress response.

Diseases	Functions Altered
• hypertension • heart disease • colitis • ulcers • irritable bowel syndrome • fibromyalgia • rheumatoid arthritis • osteoarthritis • multiple sclerosis • diabetes • thyroid disease • stroke • aneurysms • kidney disease • psoriasis • eczema • cancer • infections • aneurysm rupture	• obesity • hair loss • migraine headaches • insomnia • depression • panic attacks • the progression of HIV infection to AIDS • the emergence of latent genital herpes • the emergence of cold sores • shingles • colds and flu • wounds that won't heal • anxiety disorders • chronic fatigue syndrome • tension headaches • asthma • muscle tension • poor memory • irregular heart rhythm • short stature

Have we convinced you that Peace management is worth any effort you will need to put forth to change your mode of operation? Remember, the only purpose for inclusion of this *entire* section is to raise your consciousness that stress *is* a bad thing for your health. You get an "A" for effort entered in my grade book.

References Cited

Epel, E.S., Blackburn, E.H., Lin, J., Dhabhar, F.S., Adler, N.E., Morrow, J. D., & Cawthorn, R.M. (2004). Accelerated telomere shortening in response to life stress. Proceeding of the National Academy of Sciences, USA. Dec 7; 101 (49): 17312-5.

Guyton, A.C. & Hall, J.E. (2000). *Textbook of Medical Physiology.* 10th ed. Philadelphia: W.B. Saunders Company

Huether, S.E. & McCance (2004). *Understanding Pathophysiology.* 3rd ed. St. Louis: Mosby.

Sapolsky, R.M. (2004). *Why Zebras Don't Get Ulcers.* 3rd ed. New York: Henry Holt and Company, LLC

Please note: Several articles and text books were utilized in preparation of this section. However, only the above titles were included here because they were cited in this book. For further reading, if your interest has been captured, I would strongly suggest the book by Robert Sapolsky.

Part 6:

Summary & Future Of Peace Management

11 The Journey Has Just Begun

Here you are at the last section of the book! If you are like many of my students at the end of the Peace management course, you want more. Well, there may not be many more words left in this book, but in the big picture, things are just beginning. Now comes the creative part: applying the concepts, developing new techniques for new situations, sharing your newfound Peace with others, and beginning to enjoy the benefits of Peace.

Any one section of this book could be an entire book. The concepts have just been introduced here with the intention of allowing you to make them your own and incorporated them into the current you. The concepts will actually evolve for you as you evolve. I have witnessed this in myself. Remember back to the preface of the book, where I had a conversation with myself regarding doubting my ability to explain these concepts when I was still developing as a Peace manager. I finally said, "darn it, just sit down and write it!"

Remember, I was just like you, subjecting myself to the harmful effects of stress. I would perceive outside stimuli as stressful and respond in a very automatic, thoughtless way. I experienced health problems that have now been resolved. Through much self discipline, desire, awareness, and a bit of selfishness, I found Peace. And I am just like that dragonfly: I am NEVER going back!

Be aware that your biggest nemesis, or people who seem to block your attempts at Peace, are not only your biggest challenge, but also your biggest blessing. They provide the opportunities for you to practice Peace. They may even have served as the impetus for you to pick up this book in the first place. I am who I am because of *all* my life lessons. Now looking back, I wouldn't have turned my back on any of those opportunities to become the current me. All interactions are potentially an opportunity for growth.

The harmful effects of your stress may not be visible or immediately evident, but take my word for it, they will show up. I wish you could learn the lesson of the physical effects of stress from my most beloved pond fish, Lucille, as my son and I did. Lucille is the most beautiful of all the fish in my pond. She is a bright red and white, fancy-tail goldfish. She swims up to us and allows us to pet her. We love her to death, but we often joke about how dumb she is.

Countless times, Lucille swims into the skimmer, but cannot get out. As soon as we realize she is missing, we know exactly where to look. After we rescue her from the skimmer, she is covered with black spots from the stress. Within a day or two after being released back into the pond, her spots disappear. I wish that we humans had such obvious, visible, ugly marks on our body that would show up from stress. I don't think there is a person out there who would allow stress to dominate their life if we had such a grossly obvious and ugly reminder of its impact.

Somehow, the more subtle effects from stress we experience don't have the same impact. Often, the effects of stress on the human body are not manifested outwardly. The effects are internal and manifest themselves in potentially serious health problems. You might see:

- people with type II diabetes requiring medication to keep their blood sugar normal

- people with high blood pressure, requiring medication to keep their blood pressure normal
- people with ulcers
- people with cancer
- people with strokes
- people with heart disease
- people with headaches
- people with autoimmune diseases

just to name a few

Please realize, those health conditions are similar to Lucille's spots, just not as obviously associated in your mind. Pat your self on the back for beginning this process toward Peace.

Do not be hard on yourself for slip-ups. Even the best Peace managers need to implement stress management or anger management techniques occasionally. This is to allow you to get back to a baseline of Peace so that you may then practice Peace management. Be aware that when you are sleepy, weary, or hungry you will be more vulnerable to stress. At these times, you need to go into high protection mode and not allow anything to rob your Peace. Keep life very simple during these times.

Many of us suffer from a humor deficit. Laugh loud, laugh often, and laugh at yourself. This leaves no room for shame or guilt.

You may have noticed that the "P" in Peace is capitalized. This is not an editing error.

Lead by example and encourage those whom are interested in achieving Peace to begin an inquiry. Not only will it benefit them, but it will also make your attempt to manage Peace easier. It is very helpful to have the people close to you understand the concepts and benefits of living life from a place of Peace. As I prepare to hand over this manuscript to the editor, I have one last story for you to demonstrate the value of others in your life understanding Peace management.

When I was backing out of the driveway today, I crunched the fender of my husband's car. Luckily, even the loud noise didn't give me a charge, because I thought I had run into a mound of snow that was piled in the corner of the driveway. When I got out of my car to see if there was any damage to my car, I saw there wasn't, but I did see a big wrinkle in my husband's car. There was not a bit of a charge! I realized how proud I was of myself for that. But the best part was when I called my husband, who happens to be a car-guy. He was completely calm, which allowed me not to feel bad for not reacting with intense emotion.

Do I wish I could turn back the clock? . . . yes
Can I? . . . no
Was I aware that repair of the damage will cost money and time? . . . yes
Will stress make it cost less? . . . no
Do I realize this was not a "responsible" thing to do? . . . yes
Will stress make me feel better now? . . .no
Do I wish It didn't happen? . . . yes
Did anything good come from this? . . . yes, YES!

I had a chance to experience Peace during a situation that formerly would have caused me a great deal of stress and I got wonderful exposure to my husband's calm nature.

Because my husband is a Peace manager too and also cares about my Peace, he was very kind and supportive. I was very clear that he did not want me to experience a charge and that he knew this was an opportunity for him to demonstrate that he cared about me, my Peace, and my health. It is very beneficial when everyone in a household works to practice Peace and wants it, above all else, for everyone else in their family. You will soon see that it is what you want for everyone: your friends, neighbors, the clerks at the grocery store, and complete strangers.

When my husband got home from work this evening, he continued to maintain Peace. We even joked that the book needed a final story, so I was "blessed" with this experience for the purpose of sharing it with you. I passed! I am a successful Peace manager!

Please realize you may not be able to make others around you understand Peace management or its benefits. In the last year, I have come to accept this myself. When you "get it," you want everyone to experience it. Peace management just may not be their path, or the time might not be right. This realization of the need to let go, came to me because of a recurring dream.

I would dream that I was in an incredible place in Hawaii. In my dream, I went off on my own to find an even more incredible place. It was along a very long, lush path. The path ended at a place that was beyond description; the beauty and peace were palpable. I hurried back to have other people go back with me to experience this place.

Every time I had the dream, various people would start off with me, but they would get distracted by various activities or interests. Sometimes, I didn't even realize that they were gone until I turned to see their expression, only to discover I was alone. I would get to this place that felt like the Garden of Eden, and I would be by myself, unable to share the beauty with others.

I finally became aware of the meaning when I dreamt that I was leading two of my most skilled and delightful nursing students down the path. Like the rest, they soon turned off the path. In reality, these former nursing students were clinically two of the sharpest I have had in my years of teaching, yet they both had extreme test anxiety.

I strongly and repeatedly advocated they receive tutoring from a very reputable and successful tutor in our area before they took Boards. They both decided to go with another tutor system, because it was $50 cheaper than the one I recommended. They both failed Boards due to their extreme test anxiety. They ended up going to the tutor that I recommended at a "repeaters" cost of $1200. They both passed the second time.

I soon realized that my dream meant that even though I think I know what might benefit someone, it is up to that person to make their own decisions about the direction of their life. I have to let go. Those I have tried to help but who are not ready or willing know I will be here with open arms and an open heart should they choose to embrace Peace. I suggest the same for you. All you can do is live an exemplary life and others may absorb some of your Peace, simply by being exposed to you.

Continually evaluate your progress with Peace management. You may want to occasionally rate yourself on a scale on 1-10 to determine if you are making progress. Notice if your periods of "charge" are less intense, less frequent, and do not last as long. Notice if your baseline is more calm. And notice if you experience deeper levels of Peace.

Now it is time for your final exam. You need to go shopping at a mall on the day after Thanksgiving and make yourself purchase two things (one at an electronics superstore would get you bonus points.) And you are not allowed to go early in the morning when there are still parking spaces. If you don't have small children of your own, borrow someone else's kids. If they have a cold you get extra points. If you are able to stay in a place of Peace all day, you graduate summa cum laude from your own school of higher education. Good luck in graduate school!

Dear Peace manager,

I send you off with my best wishes for a joyful and "Peace-full" life. I want you to know that I know you. I feel your trials, struggles, triumphs, and growth. I have witnessed them in thousands. I know each person has a unique story, yet we are all the same on many levels and in many areas. That is the part of you I know without ever having met you. I know your humanness.

This ability, for humans to know humans is the part of me, that, as a nurse, allows me to begin caring for my patients in a very connected way, without ever having had the pleasure to know them before they were in my intensive care bed. Please know that as you were reading this book, you were in my prayers.

I pray that all the individuals that I work with will successfully learn to manage their Peace. If you read this book, it is your desire to have Peace. So since it is your desire, it is my desire that you will be successful.

Please take the knowledge and information from this book and apply it to all areas of your life. My hope is that you continue this application until Peace management permeates all areas of your life. Serve as a role model for Peace. Others will want to know, "what is your secret?" It is no secret: you live life from a place of Peace, which allows you to experience more joy.

I have many wishes for you, my friend:

I wish that you are able to appropriately find a strategy to manage Peace in all situations.

I wish that you serve as your own stabilizing force in all areas of your life. I wish the experience of health, well-being, joy and Peace have a profound effect on your life, relationships, and time on Earth.

I wish that by example, information, and creativity you share this in a way that allows you to transform the lives of all around you who desire Peace. I wish you a life that is full of Joy and happiness.

I wish you challenges that allow you to experience true strength, power, and self control as you maintain your Peace.

But most of all, I wish you Peace!

Many blessings on your path,
Gina Marie

I would like to let you peek in on my future plans for Peace management:

I would like everyone who wants to find Peace to have access to this information. Therefore, it will be available in various formats, including videotapes, audio books, pamphlets, seminars/workshops, and one-on-one counseling.

There is a whole second tier of books in the works. They are focused on the application of Peace management and are targeted for specific groups. They are in various stages of development and writing. For some of them, I am still in the process of putting together a team of experts. Here are some of the books under development at this time:

- *Peace Management for Children*
- A children's book for teaching Peace management
- A book to expand a teens' way of thinking
- *Peace Management for Couples*
- Peace management to replace anger management mandated by courts
- *Peace Management in the Workplace*
- *Advanced Peace Management for Personal Growth*
- *Peace Management for the Golden Years*
- *Peace Management for the Person who is Dying*
- *Peace Management During Divorce*
- *Peace Management: A Nurse's Application for Patient Care*

I also intend to create easy access for nurses and other health care professionals to learn Peace management. I plan on training and certifying facilitators to teach these courses. Frequently, my students say, "will you please come talk to my patient?" This makes me realize that others see the immediate need for implementing Peace management with patients, but do not feel skilled enough to communicate this information. My goal is to have health care providers become very comfortable with this program in their own lives, so that they may assist patients.

I encourage anyone who has the desire to research the benefits of Peace management to do so. This would help substantiate the benefits of the program. Individuals do not seem to need statistics to understand the benefits of Peace management; they are their own best source for determining the benefit. The benefit of research would be the shift in the view of society. I would cooperate with any research endeavor, including any information you need or assistance with programs. I would love to eventually establish a foundation to award grants for this type of research.

A few other areas for development will be:

- video tapes that will aid study groups to guide their week-to-week sessions
- a journal guide, as I have witnessed the most dramatic growth in students who have journaled their progress through the process

And the ideas keep coming. People who have gone through the course, both my nursing students and those in the community, frequently forward me ideas to assist others with the program. Keep the ideas coming! I would love to hear from you, too.

My web site will have continually updated information. There is also e-mail ability. The web site is:

www.peacemanagement.info

Get to know the Author

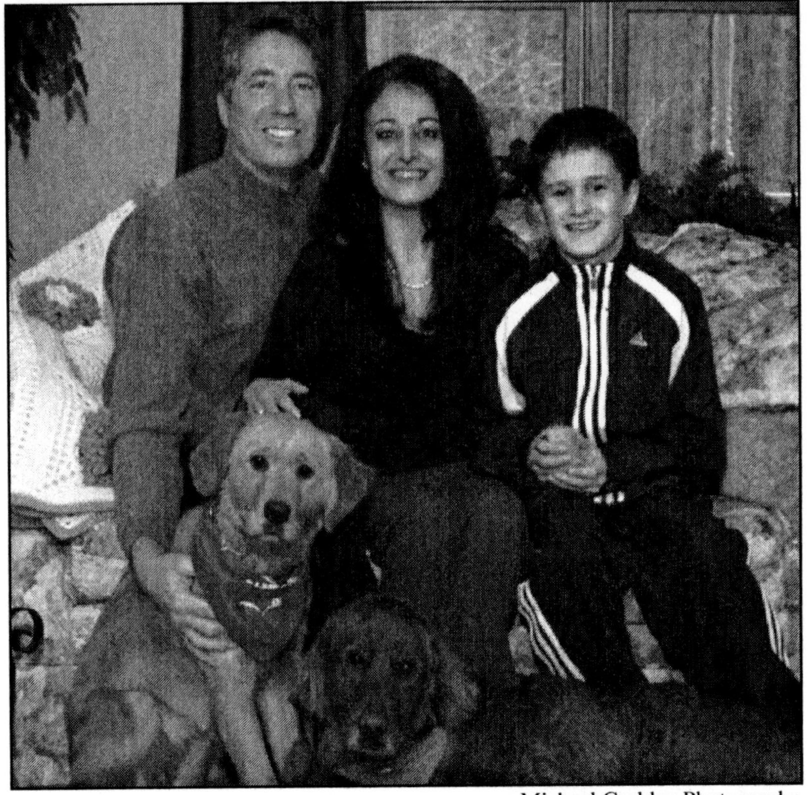

Michael Corbley Photography

I have the pleasure of introducing my colleague and best friend, Gina Marie McKee. Gina Marie has been my best friend for twenty-seven years. We worked together on a medical division of a community hospital in our pre-RN days and as RNs in an Intensive Care Unit setting for several years. Our professional paths merged many times throughout our careers, including a recent joint effort with her nursing students. Gina Marie's nursing students were on the division where I worked at a large Cleveland hospital. I had many opportunities to work with her students and enjoyed the stories they shared about the benefits of Peace management in their lives.

As her best friend, I have had the opportunity to share many life experiences with Gina Marie. I have grown tremendously and now experience Peace on a more regular basis, and witnessed an amazing transformation in Gina Marie as she became a Peace manager. The energy of Peace and joy emanate constantly from her, and she always has a positive effect on those around her. What I find most amazing is the transformation her students describe after being in Gina Marie's class for only 5 weeks. Her students have credited Peace management for varied benefits. One student told me "Peace management has saved my marriage" and another reported "now I don't freak out on exams." Gina Marie's students have even explained how Peace management has transformed whole families. The students' spouses use the phraseology of Peace management, and the students' children help their parents do a charge check.

Gina Marie's whole career has been focused on wellness. From early in her career, she was dissatisfied with the type of treatment that we, as health care providers, utilize. Even in the intensive care setting, with all our machines, medicines, and diagnostic tools, Gina Marie felt that it wasn't enough. She has witnessed the horrors that create extreme disease and illness in the human bodies of sacred souls. She has cried countless times as she has watched her beloved patients succumb to the ills of disease. Putting "band-aids" on eroded, diseased body parts was not the answer in her mind.

I am not surprised that Gina Marie's path led her to Peace management. Everything in her career pointed toward figuring out a way to make a real difference. At the community hospital where we worked together, she advanced from a nursing assistant all the way to Assistant Director of Nursing. She created a wellness and exercise program for senior citizens at a hospital. She focused on wellness in her roles as Diabetic Educator and Cardiac Rehabilitation nurse.

Gina Marie's desire to teach nursing students also stems from her desire to make a difference. Gina Marie has been an educator her entire career and has taught nursing for sixteen years. She has taught at Case Western Reserve University, Ursuline College, and Lakeland Community Colleges in northeast Ohio. She feels that many can teach the skills and tasks of a nurse, but she wants to have a much bigger impact on the next generation of nurses. When it comes to nursing, Gina Marie "gets it," and we can only hope that when we are old there will be enough nurses out there who have been impacted by the love and guidance of Gina Marie to care for us.

Professionally, Gina Marie is an educator. But her educational mission extends far beyond her professional roles. Gina Marie is a gifted teacher in all facets of her life. Essentially, she is always teaching. When she is with children she seems to be creating simple fun, but there is always some form of education going on. She also teaches by example and role modeling,

Gina Marie has had a very accomplished career in a variety of health care and university settings. But I know there would be no greater honor or satisfaction for Gina Marie than to know she may be improving the health of those whom she has touched. Helping others find health through Peace management will be the crown jewel in her career and life.

Family is very important to Gina Marie. And when I use the word "family" here, I mean it in the broadest sense. Gina Marie has a very large "adopted family" of which my children, Kyle and Jackie (Gina Marie's "adopted" nephew and niece), and I are a part. All who cross the path of Gina Marie are taken in by her genuine love, concern, and care. In fact, all of her nursing students, are part of her family. Many students and former students say she nurtures them through difficult times as well as personal and professional development. They know she really loves them.

Gina Marie is also blessed with a wonderful family of origin, who mean the world to her. In fact, as she began to witness the ills that were beginning to fall on her family and herself as a result of the stress of a divorce, she finally said "this is enough." She began a different way of life which now has a name: Peace management.

Gina Marie has a twelve year old son, Grant, whom she admires, loves, and feels intense pride in. Her husband is Gary, someone she has been friends with for twenty-five years. They share a fun and loving relationship. Her parents are loving and supportive, and her extended family provides a sense of love and belonging.

Life has not always been easy for Gina Marie, but because of her growth through all her life's lessons, she is an incredible culmination of her experiences. I hope you get a sense of this woman through reading her book, or having an opportunity to meet or work with her as she takes Peace management to the world. Gina Marie's hard won wisdom has yielded great benefits for me. I trust it will for you, too.

Kim Patton-Schroeder, BSN, RN